RESPIRATORY DISEASE

D0569208

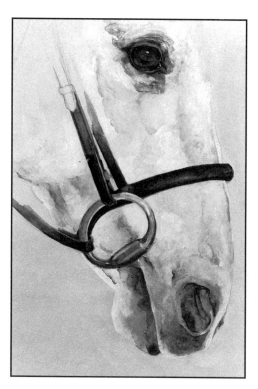

RESPIRATORY DISEASE

Peter Gray

MVB, MRCVS

J. A. Allen
London

British Library Cataloguing in Publication Data
A catalogue record for this book is available from the British Library

ISBN 0 85131 570 4

Published in Great Britain in 1994 by
J. A. Allen & Company Limited
1 Lower Grosvenor Place
London SW1W 0EL

© Peter Gray 1994

No part of this book may be reproduced or transmitted in any way or by any means, electronic, or mechanical, including photocopy, recording, or any information storage and retrieval system, without permission in writing from the publishers. All rights reserved.

Production editor: Bill Ireson
Illustrator: Maggie Raynor
Series designer: Nancy Lawrence
Printed in Great Britain by The Bath Press, Avon

To Emily and Celina

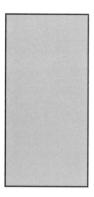

Contents

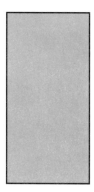

Acknowledgements

For her assistance in editing the manuscript, especially in regard to viral diseases, I would like to express my gratitude to Dr J. A. Mumford, BSc., PhD., of the Animal Health Trust, Newmarket. And, for his help with the bacterial section of the book, I thank Mr N. Chanter, BSc., PhD., also of the Animal Health Trust.

My thanks also go to Averil Opperman for her support and help in the editorial work.

My special thanks to Maggie Raynor, for her excellent artwork, to Bill Ireson, for his production editing, to series designer Nancy Lawrence, and to my publishers.

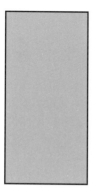

Introduction

The purpose of this book is to provide up-to-date information on equine respiratory disease, for anyone with an interest, whether professional or personal, in the subject.

Such information is often complex and necessarily has sometimes to be presented in a language that poses difficulties for those with no medical background. However, for anyone involved with horses, the importance of having some knowledge of the technical aspects of disease cannot be underestimated. Technical definitions are a part of standard sales terms. They also matter in the routine conduct of law. It is important, therefore, that horseowners should have some understanding of specific respiratory conditions which they are likely to encounter (in sales catalogues for instance) and what they mean in relation to airway obstruction and soundness.

It is to be hoped that *Respiratory Disease* will become a standard textbook for non-veterinarians, marrying the latest in scientific knowledge with the practical everyday information of clinical practice. Its ultimate aim is to bring to the horseman and horsewoman solid advice on the management of respiratory disease which is an essential adjunct to any form of therapy.

Understanding the respiratory system is particularly important because of the dynamic nature of the horse and the principle purpose, athleticism, for which it is used today. As this system is the medium of gaseous exchange between living animal and surrounding environment, it is responsible for providing all oxygen requirements of the body, including the musculature during locomotion. It also allows the removal of carbon dioxide to the exterior. At exercise, without adequate oxygen, there is reduced capacity to perform - even when the deprivation is only partial. The influence of such shortage is critical to any competing horse.

Oxygen deficiency occurs in horses and is recognised as an expression of functional respiratory disease, including infection, or as a secondary consequence of diseases of other organs such as the heart and blood. For example, heart disease can often result in lowered tissue oxygenisation because of failure to circulate the blood; and, as a different example, nitrite poisoning can cause a reduction of the blood's capacity to carry oxygen.

In the United Kingdom and Ireland today there is a high incidence of primary respiratory disease in horses. This directly affects the interests of many people and has a significant economic influence on the equine industry. Infection occurs because the respiratory system is a common portal of entry for foreign matter into the body, including organisms such as bacteria and viruses. There is also a high incidence of non-infectious respiratory disease, such as chronic obstructive pulmonary disease (COPD), which has allergic and other causes. In reality, much of this disease reflects errors that are being made in the controllable aspects of horse management, including the environment of the stable.

Low-grade viral infection would appear to have increased remarkably in modern times. This has been due in part to an increase in horse numbers but also reflects the new styles of management which a growing horse population requires, especially in the areas of breeding and sport. Increased competition and wider international transport for racing and breeding purposes now allows for a more distant spread of infectious organisms and the added stress of travel can make individual horses more susceptible to attack. Once infected, these horses introduce their germs to the varying populations with which they come into contact.

Both environment and management influence the establishment of disease and have a profound affect on the manner in which resistance and immune mechanisms help horses to withstand challenge. It is vital to the control of infection that these processes be understood; also that the character and nature of organisms be appreciated, and interference made at the appropriate time and place, in order to break the cycle they can establish.

The present day approach to control appears to be for the reduction of disease by vaccination alone. Not only is this approach unsatisfactory because of the quality of present vaccines, but it would be foolish in the extreme to believe that even effective vaccines will stem the problem as we now know it. To suggest this is to fail to appreciate the principles involved; unless we broaden our understanding the lessons to be learned will be even more painful than those of the past. Simply expressed, there is a growing pool of disease agents that we recognise and an increasing, susceptible, horse population. Unless we appreciate the real significance of this, disease will prosper and human interest will be made to suffer.

Finally, there is a changing temper internationally in the attitudes of equine sales companies to the problems of mechanical diseases of the upper respiratory tract. The best known of these diseases is ILH - or, as it is more commonly referred to, 'whistling and roaring' (its medical description is idiopathic laryngeal hemiplegia).

The broadening of understanding regarding conditions of the larynx has come with the advent of the fibreoptic endoscope, but this understanding rests largely within the professional sphere. It is becoming increasingly important that owners, trainers and others should have a ready reference to these problems, all of which are within the remit of this book.

On the other hand, it is not the purpose of the book to take the reader into the sphere of advanced clinical technology. While it is important to encourage the horse owner to achieve a higher standard of management and observation, there is a line beyond which an animal must be entrusted to expert and specialist care; that line is drawn between information and responsibility and this book sits astride it, where it can best benefit layman and veterinary surgeon alike.

Peter Gray

Author Note
I have used everyday and common terms when naming parts of the horse. In veterinary practice, of course, technical names are used for greater accuracy of definition. When it will aid the reader, therefore, I have occasionally used both in the text and index.

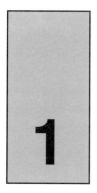

Anatomy of the Respiratory System

For practical purposes, the respiratory system begins at the nostrils and continues through the nasal passages to the nasopharynx, then through the larynx to the trachea, on to the bronchi, bronchioles and finally to the alveoli of the lungs where gas exchange occurs between inspired air and circulating blood.

The respiratory system. The lungs here are fully expanded, though when at rest the horse's full lung capacity is not used

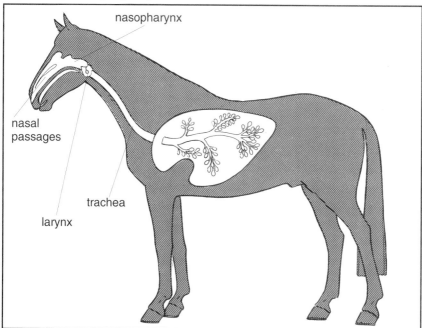

Besides these main channels of airflow, there are structures such as the paranasal sinuses and gutteral pouches which are classified as part of the respiratory system, as well as the turbinate bones that divide the nasal passages and offer a wide membranous surface for contact with incoming air.

Nostrils

The nostril, the entrance to the nasal chamber, is a large somewhat oval opening bounded on either side by wings (*alae*). These wings meet above and below to form the extremities, called commissures, the upper being narrow, the lower wide and rounded.

Cartilage provides support for the rims of the nostrils and prevents them closing during inspiration. If a finger is introduced upwards, from below the upper commissure, it will enter the false nostril, a pocket formed on the upper inside of the nostril. This is about 10cm deep and lined by a continuation of the skin and not by the mucous membrane which covers the inner surface of the nasal passages.

The function of the false nostril is to filter off dirt that comes into its path. It is also noteworthy as the site of origin of high-blowing in horses. This noise, which is not abnormal, may occur during the expiratory phase of the breathing cycle.

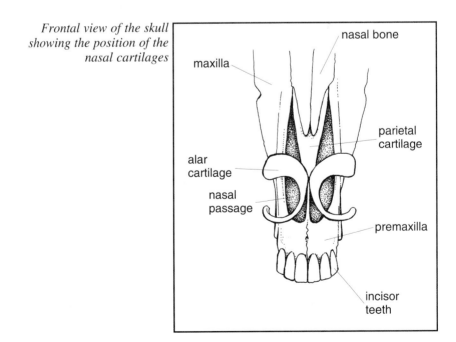

Frontal view of the skull showing the position of the nasal cartilages

maxilla

nasal bone

parietal cartilage

alar cartilage

nasal passage

premaxilla

incisor teeth

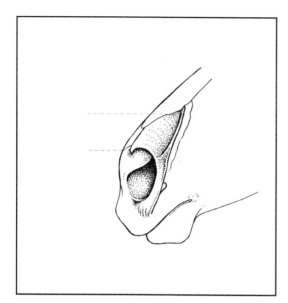

*The nostril dilated; the upper outline (*broken lines*) showing the extent of the false nostril*

However, high blowing may cause confusion when horses are being tried for their wind by making it difficult to distinguish abnormal sounds. There is a small circular hole, about 5cm from the lower commissure, formed as if a piece of skin has been punched out; the hole is the lower opening of the nasolacrimal duct through which tears drain from the eye to the nose. Just beyond this hole the skin is continued by pink mucous membrane which lines the rest of the nasal passages.

Muscular action on the cartilages permits the nostrils to dilate and contract. They also dilate by the forcible expiration of air during the act of snorting.

Nasal Passages

The bony boundaries of the nasal passages are as described below.
1)   The nasal bones form the roof of the passage.
2)   The maxillary bones form the walls.
3)   The hard palate forms the floor.
4)   The ethmoturbinates form the back wall just above the entrance into the nasopharynx.
5)   The nasal septum separates the nasal passages of either side.

These boundaries enclose the closely-rolled turbinate bones (*conchae*), situated two on either side of the nasal septum.

Nasal Bones

The nasal bones are bilateral and triangular in shape with their bases uniting with the frontal and lachrymal bones, while their apices form the sharp, pointed nasal peak. The two bones lie side-by-side and in the young animal are mainly united by cartilaginous material which becomes converted into bone later in life. Each is convex from side-to-side on its outer surface and concave on its inner.

Maxillae

The maxillae are the principle bones of the upper jaw and carry the upper cheek teeth. They are easily felt on the outer surface of the face. The nasal surface is concave and forms the greater part of the outside wall of the nasal cavity.

Hard Palate

The palatine bones and processes of the maxilla and premaxilla together help to form the bony floor of the nasal cavity (and roof of the mouth) known as the hard palate.

The bones of the skull

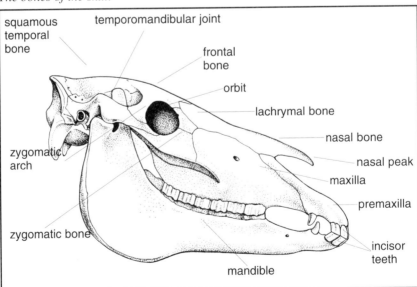

Ethmoturbinates

At the back of the nasal cavity the nasal passages communicate with the nasopharynx through the *choanae* or posterior nares, which are separated by a single bone, the vomer.

The ethmoturbinate area, above the posterior nares, is highly vascular and is closely associated with the sense of smell.

Turbinate Bones (*Conchae*)

The nasal passages contain the two tightly-rolled turbinate bones, the purpose of which is to extend the amount of surface membrane to which incoming air is exposed.

Between them the turbinates divide each nasal passage into three channels: the dorsal meatus, the middle meatus and the ventral meatus. The dorsal meatus is closed at its posterior end and it conducts air to the olfactory area - the region of smell. The middle meatus falls between the two turbinates and has at its posterior end the opening of one of the facial sinuses, the maxillary sinus. The ventral meatus is by far the largest and is the channel along which stomach tubes and endoscopes are normally passed in clinical practice. It is the direct channel between the nostrils and pharynx.

Cross-section of the skull showing the position of the turbinate bones

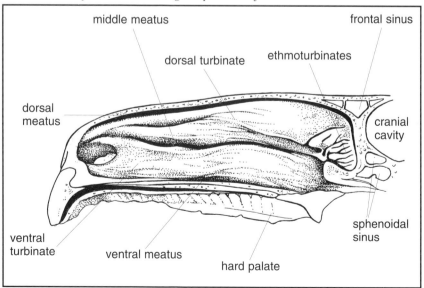

Nasal Mucous Membrane

A thick, highly vascular lining, the nasal mucous membrane is firmly attached to the underlying bones. It is continuous with the lining of the paranasal sinuses and that of the pharynx behind. The dimensions of the lower (or ventral) meatus can be increased in fast exercise by constriction of the vessels in this membrane.

Nasopharynx

The nasopharynx is the backward continuation of the horse's nasal passage, situated above the soft palate at the back of the mouth and allowing communication between the posterior nares and the larynx. Its long axis is downward and backward and it is about 15cm in length.

Soft Palate

The soft palate is an oblique, valve-like curtain which separates the mouth cavity from the pharynx. Its anterior (oral) surface looks downwards and forwards and is covered with mucous membrane continuous with that of the hard palate. Its posterior (pharyngeal) surface is covered by a mucous membrane that is continuous with the nasal passages.

Owing to its length - the free border of the soft palate contacts the epiglottis of the larynx - the pharynx is closed from the mouth except during the passage of food or drink to the oesophagus. The manner of this contact is important - as a virtual seal is formed which especially protects the respiratory tract from aspiration of food material passing between the mouth and oesophagus (gullet). The epiglottis also plays a part in this process.

The large size and functional anatomy of the soft palate explains why mouth breathing is not natural to the horse; also why it has difficulty vomiting. If vomiting does occur the ejected matter escapes usually through the nostrils.

The pharyngeal wall is occupied by the diffuse tonsil, a structure which has particular importance as the site of entry of many organisms into the body - such as that which causes strangles (*Streptococcus equi*).

The purpose of the pharynx is to allow passage of food into the oesophagus from the mouth without interference with breathing and to allow air from the nasal passages to enter the larynx without any similar hindrance.

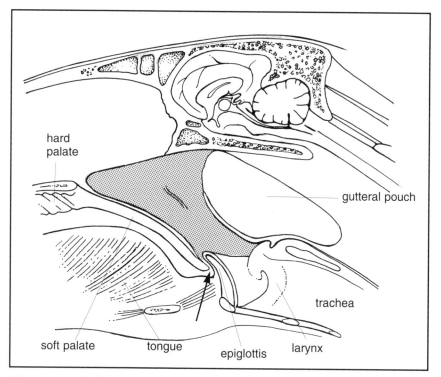

The extent of the nasopharynx (tinted area at centre) *with the soft palate* (arrowed) *beneath the epiglottis, the airway open*

The division of these purposes is achieved by the soft palate, the epiglottis and the tongue. Under normal circumstances, when the horse is not swallowing, the soft palate almost surrounds the larynx, sitting beneath the epiglottis. When the horse swallows, the tongue presses backwards, the epiglottis closes off the entrance to the larynx and the soft palate is moved dorsally so that food can enter the oesophagus and not be returned into the nasal passages. As soon as the food has crossed the pharynx the soft palate returns to close the seal and breathing resumes.

Also present in the nasopharynx are the paired openings to the gutteral pouches.

Paranasal Sinuses

The comparatively large size of the horse's skull results from the evolution of the substantial eating apparatus the horse needs to survive in

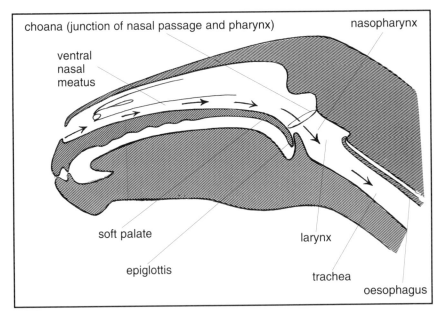

Air travelling (arrowed, above) *along the ventral nasal meatus, through the nasopharynx and larynx into the trachea. The mouth is closed off from the pharynx by the position of the soft palate in front of the epiglottis. In swallowing* (below) *backward movement of the tongue presses the epiglottis back to close off the larynx and lifts the soft palate to prevent entry of food material into the nasal chamber (passages), thus protecting the respiratory system in both directions*

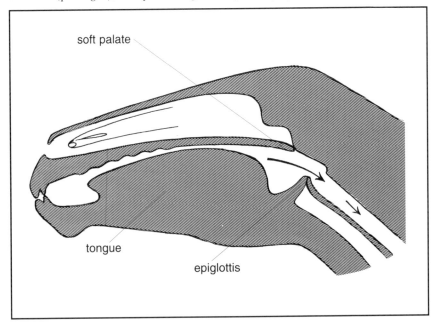

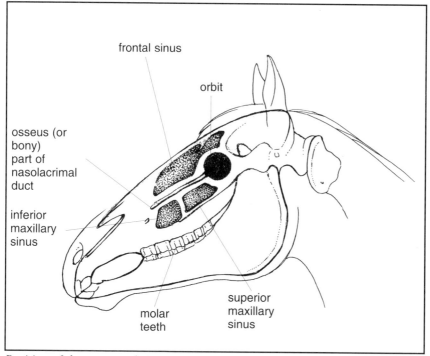

Position of the paranasal sinuses relative to the orbit and molar teeth

nature. Had this apparatus been achieved by extra bone deposition, it would have increased the weight of the horse's head excessively. Therefore, evolution enlarged the bones by including air cavities within them so that surface area was increased without any great increase in volume, or weight, of the whole.

There are a number of sinuses in each half of the head, namely the frontal, superior and inferior maxillary, and sphenopalatine (consisting of sphenoidal and palatine parts) sinuses at the base of the cranium.

The sinuses fill, or at least change, some part of their air content during expiration. They are lined by a continuation of the mucous membrane of the nasal passage and are readily involved in the course of nasal infections. In the horse at least they have no recognised function other than to provide the head with size and contour. They have no part in the horse's sense of smell.

Gutteral Pouches

The gutteral pouches are structures found only in the horse family and

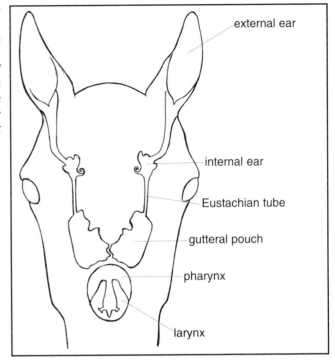

The relationships of the pharynx, gutteral pouch and internal ear. Each gutteral pouch communicates directly with the pharynx

exist as dilatations of the Eustachian tubes, the thin membranous channels that connect the nasopharynx with each middle ear.

Each gutteral pouch has a capacity of about 300ml and the purpose of the Eustachian tube, though uncertain, is probably to equalise air pressure on either side of the tympanic membrane of the middle ear, the eardrum.

During expiration, or swallowing, the gutteral pouches are thought to fill with air. During swallowing, the openings of the Eustachian tubes on the roof of the pharynx become patent and the soft palate contacts the pharyngeal roof behind them, preventing the passage of any food material upwards at this time.

Larynx

The larynx is a short tubular structure situated between the pharynx and trachea - the passage leading from the nasal chambers to the lungs.

Often called the voice-box, the larynx contains the horse's vocal cords. Its primary purpose is to regulate the flow of air during respiration and to prevent the aspiration of foreign material, such as food.

It is made up of five cartilages articulated together: the cricoid, thyroid

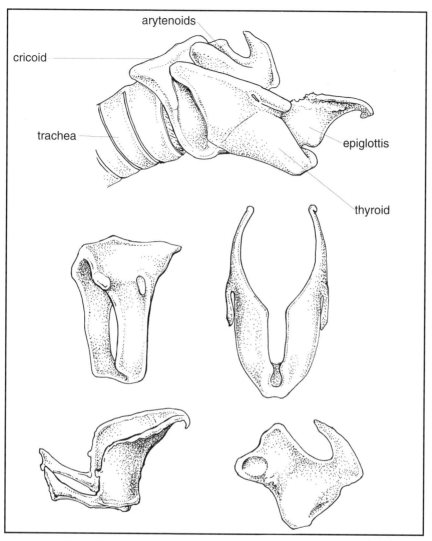

Anatomy of the horse's throat: larynx (top)*; cricoid cartilage* (centre, left)*; epiglottic cartilage* (bottom, left)*; thyroid cartilage, ventral view* (centre, right)*; and left arytenoid cartilage* (bottom right)

and epiglottis are single cartilages, the arytenoid cartilage is paired. These cartilages serve as attachment areas for muscles which open and close the glottis (the opening into the larynx). The epiglottis rests in the median plane and is the most anterior of the cartilages, projecting in front of the glottis.

Paralysis of the muscles activating one of the two arytenoid cartilages, most commonly that of the left side, causes partial obstruction of the airway when air is passing inwardly. This occurs in the condition which the layman calls 'whistling and roaring', but which the veterinary profession more accurately names as ILH (idiopathic laryngeal hemiplegia).

Hyoid Bone

The hyoid bone is situated at the base of the horse's tongue. It is a complex structure that resembles a child's swing with the body of the hyoid

The hyoid apparatus (top); *and its relationship to the larynx* (bottom)

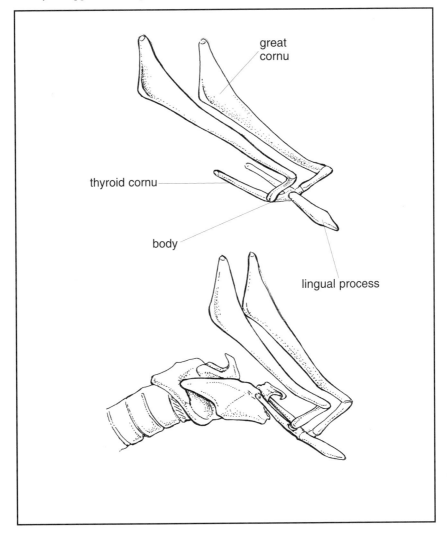

being the seat. The body is also joined up with the larynx and the root of the tongue. The hyoid therefore serves as an important area of attachment of tongue, pharyngeal and laryngeal muscles, and also serves to suspend the larynx in the ventral part of the throat.

Trachea

The trachea consists of 48 to 60 incomplete cartilaginous rings. Each ring measures between 2cm and 3cm from front to back and some 5cm to 6cm in diameter. The trachea is the tube that connects the larynx with the bronchi of the lungs. It is freely palpable on the lower surface of the neck where it lies above two thin muscles. The jugular veins, carotid arteries and the vagus, sympathetic and recurrent laryngeal nerves lie to either side of it and the oesophagus lies above and to the left.

The trachea is lined by a type of epithelium that contains cilia, formed so as to sweep inhaled foreign matter upwards to the exterior.

Bronchi

The trachea divides into two bronchi at the level of about the fifth or sixth rib above the base of the heart. Each bronchus communicates with a lung in which it divides into innumerable smaller bronchioles. These gradually reduce in size as they approach the alveoli of the lungs in which air exchange occurs. The larger bronchioles are supported by cartilage; those smaller than 1mm are not.

Lungs

There are two lungs, right and left, which rest within the chest cavity above the heart. They are adapted to the shape of the chest wall, although the right lung is larger than the left. In the living state, the lungs fill the chest cavity around the heart. If air enters the chest cavity, perhaps through a puncture wound, the lung on the affected side is likely to collapse.

The tissue of the lungs is soft, spongy and very elastic. Under normal circumstances, healthy lung tissue tested in the laboratory will float in water. Where it is consolidated - as might happen, for example, if taken from an animal that had died from pneumonia - the tissue will sink. The

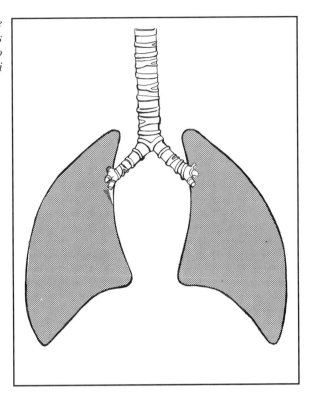

The lungs, showing the trachea and its bifurcation into two bronchi

colour of a healthy lung is normally pale pink, though this may vary with the quantity of blood retained within its tissues. In disease, depending on the type of condition involved, colour varies from pale pink (in some chronic non-infectious conditions) to deep blue or purple (in pneumonia).

The front of the inner surface of each lung is shaped so as to accommodate the heart in the centre of the chest cavity.

The blood supply to the lungs is of great importance; on the one hand it must allow for normal nourishment of the lung tissues themselves and, on the other, venous blood must be brought to the alveolar surface for oxygenation. This arrangement allows for the release of carbon dioxide as well as the collection of oxygen to be distributed to body tissues.

Pleura

The pleura are thin transparent membranes that cover the lining of the chest wall (the parietal pleura) and the substance of the lungs themselves (the pulmonary or visceral pleura). Between these two distinct surfaces, the pleural sac contains a clear serous fluid which helps to lubricate the

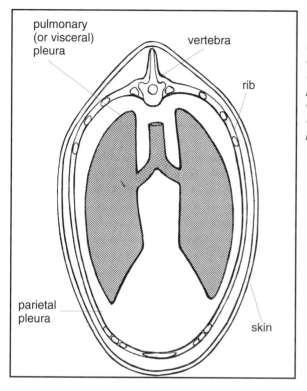

pulmonary (or visceral) pleura

vertebra

rib

parietal pleura

skin

Cross-section of the thorax, showing how the pleura form the outer covering of the lungs (pulmonary pleura) and the inner covering of the thoracic wall (parietal pleura)

surfaces and facilitate expansion and contraction of the lungs during breathing.

Diaphragm

The diaphragm forms the posterior wall of the chest cavity and separates it from the abdomen. A thin muscular organ, the diaphragm, along with the muscles of the thorax, is a vital part of the horse's respiratory system.

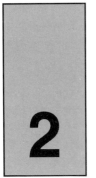

2 Physiology of the Respiratory Tract

The purpose of respiration is the exchange of gases between animal and environment. Respiration is the most intimate means by which animal life co-exists with nature, as the requirement for oxygen is immediate and ongoing. Deprivation of oxygen will result in death quicker than that of any other normal body requirement. The blood transports oxygen to the tissues continually and this allows the normal chemical processes of the body to operate.

Air entering the respiratory tract of the horse is first influenced by the warming effect of the epithelial covering of the nasal passages and the large surface area they offer through the medium of the turbinate bones. This protects the more delicate tissues deeper down from the possible harmful effects of air inhaled at temperatures below that which is compatible with life.

The upper tract is designed in such a way that there is a natural restriction to incoming airflow at the nostrils and larynx, but these are capable of being dilated by muscular action, thus creating a capacity for greater intake at increased exercise rates. The nostrils dilate, the mucous membranes of the upper tract constrict, and the larynx is brought into a more dynamic position by muscle contraction and head elevation; all of which tends to make the tract more streamlined and allows for greater volumes of air to be inspired as the need arises. This is a very important point as excessive head flexion can inhibit air intake at faster paces leading to dynamic problems within the airway.

On inhalation, the pressure exerted in the chest is negative relative to atmospheric pressure, but it is positive on exhalation. This is simply understood: as with human lungs, air is drawn into the horse's lungs by suction. Inhalation requires muscular activity, provided by the rib muscles and diaphragm, and exhalation is largely passive above a certain level of emptying, called the functional residual capacity (FRC). Beyond this level, muscular activity, provided by the abdominal muscles, is required to expel more air.

From the bronchi onwards, the air channels in the horse's lungs grow smaller, first dividing into bronchioles, and ending in terminal globules that contain alveoli which are thin walled and in very close contact with circulating blood. At this level there is only a minimal cell depth between air and blood, and gases are exchanged without restriction provided no disease is present.

The resting airflow of a disease-free horse measures about 4 litres per second. In exercise, this measurement can be increased to as much as 75 litres per second. It therefore follows that the resting lung is not using all available ventilation space.

Detail of lung anatomy showing the arrangement that leads to the alveoli

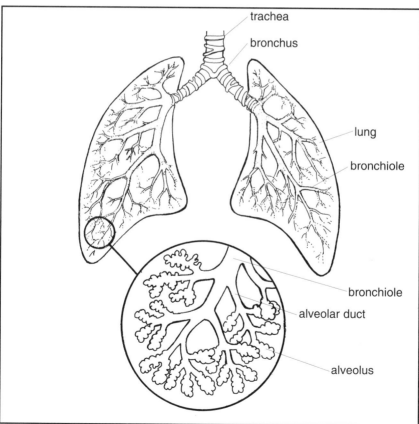

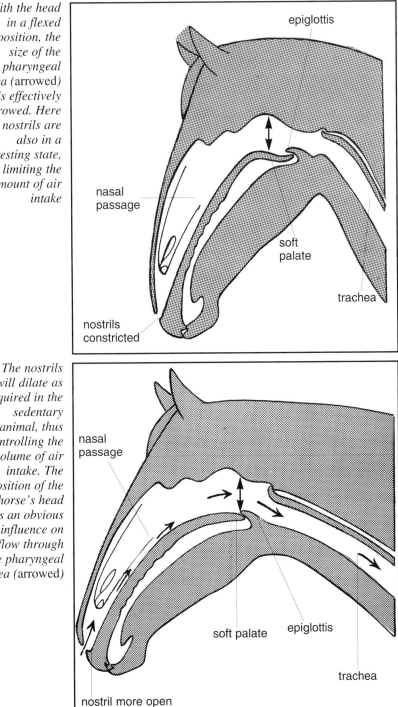

With the head in a flexed position, the size of the pharyngeal area (arrowed) is effectively narrowed. Here the nostrils are also in a resting state, limiting the amount of air intake

epiglottis

nasal passage

soft palate

trachea

nostrils constricted

The nostrils will dilate as required in the sedentary animal, thus controlling the volume of air intake. The position of the horse's head has an obvious influence on airflow through the pharyngeal area (arrowed)

nasal passage

soft palate

epiglottis

trachea

nostril more open

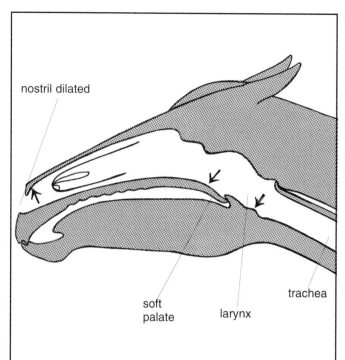

nostril dilated

soft
palate

larynx

trachea

At the gallop, the horse's head is extended and the nostrils are dilated, allowing maximum airflow to the lungs. Note the streamlining of the soft palate, larynx and trachea

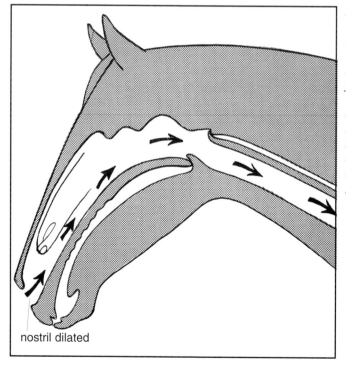

nostril dilated

As more air is required, the nostrils dilate in an animal at rest suffering from respiratory disease. The horse's head may also be extended where the demand is great

The total surface area for gas exchange is very considerable and is esti-mated to be in the region of many hundreds of square metres of alveolar tissue.

The normal resting lung, therefore, does not expand or contract fully, so that there is a residual volume of air which is not expelled. The FRC is the amount of air left in the horse's lungs at the end of resting exhalation. The normal tidal volume (average breathing volume) in a horse at rest, as stat-ed earlier, is about 4 litres of air per second. The inspired volume is greater than the expired volume because more oxygen is taken up than carbon dioxide released from the body.

In a horse at rest, the amount of air available in the trachea, bronchi and bronchioles (i.e. the air not expelled) may be as much as 70 per cent of that inhaled. Therefore only 30 per cent is involved in alveolar ventilation at rest.

The total lung capacity is reached at the end of inhalation and will be maximal when a horse is fully extended, as in the later parts of a race or competition. After competing, it is simple to see that the animal is using full available lung capacity during recovery, dilating its nostrils while breathing in and contracting its abdominal muscles strongly on expiration.

Elasticity and Compliance

The natural ability to stretch and recoil (elasticity) and elastic resistance to ventilation (compliance) are important characteristics of lung tissue and vital to the normal processes of ventilation. These characteristics are often lost where there is disease and result in increased respiratory effort and rate in order to achieve adequate oxygen intake. Generally, infection results in a loss of functional air space through consolidation of normal tissues and collapse or blockage of air passages. This inevitably reduces lung space for gas exchange.

Surfactant

A surface acting agent, surfactant reduces surface tension. It contributes to the elastic properties of lung tissue, helping to maintain alveolar stabil-ity and preventing atelectasis (the collapsed or airless state of the lung). Surfactant makes breathing easier by increasing compliance and protect-ing the delicate cells that line the alveoli. It acts at the air/liquid interface and is often missing from the lungs of immature foals, thereby causing

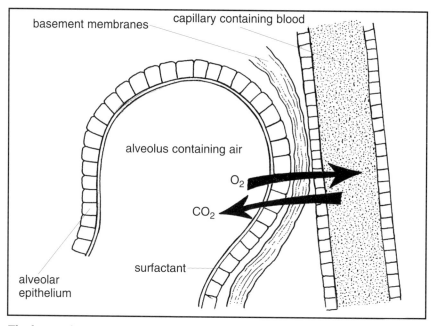

The layers that exist between the alveolar air and the capillary blood as oxygen pass into the red blood cells and carbon dioxide is released into the air

collapse of lung tissue and varying degrees of respiratory distress. Surfactant is also vital in the fight against infection.

It is essential in normal respiration, either at rest or during periods of activity, that inhaled air should match blood flow in the lungs - otherwise oxygen intake will not meet body demands. What this means in practice is that the air intake must be adequate and must reach the functioning areas of the lungs.

The upper areas of the lungs are more distended and less compliant as a rule and there is normally a preferential ventilation of lower areas.

In the alveoli, oxygen must pass through a series of barriers to reach the blood: surfactant; alveolar epithelium (surface cells); basement membrane (underlying supporting tissues); and capillary endothelium (the wall of the capillary, or minute blood vessel).

Oxygen Transfer

In the blood, oxygen combines with haemoglobin in the red cells. During exercise, there is an increased blood flow to the lungs and an increase in total circulating blood volume. These increases are due to mobilisation of

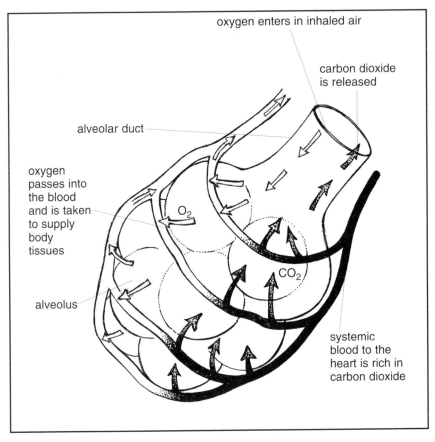

Blood flow and gas exchange in the lung

a reserve of blood cells stored in the spleen - the splenic blood reserve - with a consequent increase in red blood cells and haemoglobin. In this way, more oxygen is transported quickly. At tissue level, oxygen is released from the red blood cells and used for basic chemical processes that are vital to life.

Control of Respiration

Normal breathing is controlled centrally from the brain through the peripheral nerves. These nerves supply the muscles of respiration. Also nerve receptors in blood vessels, the lungs, trachea and bronchi respond to chemical and mechanical changes to increase or decrease respiration as the body requires it.

Coughing is caused by the stimulation of nerve receptors which are exposed as a result of tissue damage in disease.

Respiratory Mucus

The respiratory tract is covered by a double layer of mucus, which consists of sol and gel elements; this whole layer is propelled towards the pharynx by the ciliated cells of the surface membrane. It is by this means that inhaled particles are caught and expelled from the inner air passages, ideally within moments of being deposited there.

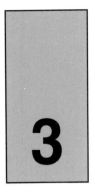

3 | Defence Against Disease

There are positive steps we can take to reduce infection, just as we can also invite disease through inadvertently failing to know the nature of the animal or appreciate the manner in which organisms invade.

The respiratory system is the most common portal of entry for viruses into the body, which means that their spread is assisted by discharges and infectious airborne material.

In this chapter we discuss the disease fighting mechanisms of the respiratory system and how it defends itself from invasion by foreign matter, be that mechanical or infectious.

Mucociliary Escalator

The horse's defences against disease are complex and form a continuing battlefront that starts at the nostrils and extends through to the blood and down into the substance of body cells.

Externally, the small hairs which line the entrances to the horse's nasal passages act as filters to foreign material entering in inhaled air. This filtering continues down along the respiratory tract, where hairs are replaced by hair-like extensions of the surface cells - the cilia. These trap dirt or organisms which reach them, and their protection extends almost to the alveoli of the lungs. Because of the mucus excreted by glands in the same membranes, this dirt is trapped and removed to the outside through a wave-like motion of the surface which simply sweeps foreign matter before it.

The mechanism to effect this motion is the mucociliary escalator and it

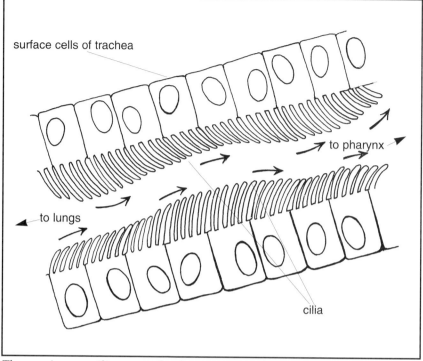

surface cells of trachea

to pharynx

to lungs

cilia

The respiratory cilia sweep foreign matter to the exterior, with a wave-like motion

is capable of returning inhaled contaminants to the surface within minutes of entry into the body.

Chemical Defences

Thus far, the defences mentioned are simply those of the mechanical, first-line protection. The second line consists of chemical defences, substances such as lysozyme interferon, interleukin, complement, and so on. These are naturally occurring substances having a direct effect on foreign matter that gains access within the body. Thus, lysozyme attacks and destroys organisms with which it comes into contact. It occurs in many body tissues and is particularly concentrated in saliva and tears.

Other substances, for example interleukin and interferon (a natural body product that inhibits growth and causes virus destruction, interferon is increasingly important as a drug in virus diseases) combine to precipitate fever by acting on the temperature regulating centre of the brain; the combination therefore acts as a defensive mechanism designed to kill organisms. Fever marks the end of the incubation period in generalised infections.

Complement is another natural defensive substance which is also used in laboratory diagnosis of viral and bacterial diseases.

The basophil cells (a variety of white blood cell, or leucocyte) contain histamine, which, when released, summon eosinophils to areas of inflammation. Eosinophils, in turn, have a critical part to play in the fight against particular types of inflammation.

Scavanger cells of the tissues (macrophages) summon other white blood cells (lymphocytes), through chemical means, to initiate immune responses and trigger inflammation.

White Blood Cells and Phagocytosis

The next defence line is held by a number of different white blood cell types and macrophages that take organisms into their substance and destroy them (phagocytosis). Here, they are aided by the effect of the chemicals already mentioned.

In the horse there are 1,000 red blood cells (RBC) for every white blood cell (WBC). The white blood cells are summoned to areas where they are needed, in injury or disease, as a result of chemical reactions, while the red blood cells are involved in oxygen and carbon dioxide transport and therefore are not directly involved in disease control.

Macrophages

Macrophages exist in blood and tissue fluids and their sole purpose is to envelop and destroy foreign material.

However, while this action is normally effective, infection depends on an organism overcoming defences, and it can happen that the defence cells are overcome. The result is immediate spread of the offending organism and, very probably, the establishment of infection.

The white blood cells try to limit the spread of infection beyond this point, and the offending organism is attacked wherever it is found - in lymph glands, liver, even within the circulation. The white blood cells involved in the defence include neutrophils, monocytes and lymphocytes (lymphocytes being unique in this group in not being phagocytic).

If the battle is lost at this stage, a virus may thrive and set up infection by multiplying in profusion, bursting out of its host cell and spilling into

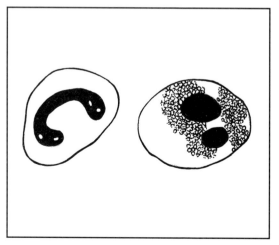

Red blood cell: in all mammals red blood cells do not have a nucleus and are in the shape of biconcave discs

Lymphocyte (left), *small, with darkly-staining nucleus; and* (right), *monocyte with kidney-shaped nucleus*

Neutrophil (left), *with a lobulated nucleus; and* (right) *eosinophil, with tightly-packed granules which may obscure the nucleus*

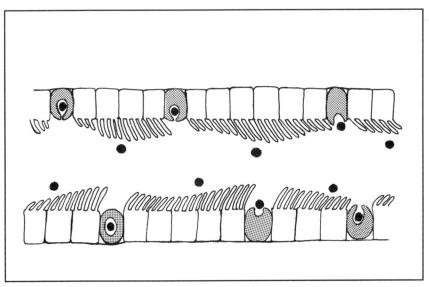

Scavenger cells in respiratory epithelium ingesting foreign particles

general circulation. The host's immune system now comes into play, bringing with it antibodies and other chemicals to support the defence.

Immunity

The immune system is the final line of defence. Immunity is active or passive, natural or acquired. What this means is that there are certain types of immunity an individual is born with, while other types develop from exposure to infection.

Active immunity is that which occurs after infection. It may have a life-long effect or it may be short-lived, as in some virus diseases. Passive immunity is that which is passively transferred from one subject to another; for example, colostrum bestows passive immunity on the foal, without which it finds it very hard to survive in its new environment. This protection lasts until the foal can develop its own immunity.

Immunity is a subject of great complexity, but is a means that is used, through vaccination, to defend animals against known infections. Vaccination against tetanus (a bacterial infection) is very effective, while against influenza (a virus) it is sometimes disappointing.

In many virus infections, the causative virus increases virulence as an epidemic builds up. Such growth allows for the development of altered varieties of virus, through mutation, against which the body will have little, or reduced, immunity. This accounts for vaccine failure as well as the prospect of new and more serious symptoms being seen.

Following infection, viruses react with defensive cells and trigger a whole range of events which result in immune responses in future infections with the same or closely related organisms. This usually results in the destruction of subsequent invaders within phagocytic cells.

Lymphocyte cells produce antibodies in lymph nodes and other lymphoid tissues; the antibodies can destroy viruses and prevent bacteria from attaching to tissue surfaces.

Resistance and Disease

Resistance is, to an extent, an expression of health. It decides the outcome of infectious disease challenge. It is, too, a measure of the health of natural tissues, of defensive mechanisms and of even the strength of cell membranes (which, for example, is reduced in Vitamin C deficiency). Resistance can be affected by age, nutrition, exposure, environment, temperature, stress, and so on.

The quantity of virus has a vital influence on the establishment of disease, as also has virulence. Together with resistance it is these factors which influence the severity of infection and the duration of illness.

It is a tribute to the effectiveness of defensive systems that our animals so seldom die of infection. Lowered resistance is a common problem with lethal infections of foals, although the overall mortality rate in equine infectious disease is thankfully low.

Particle Size and Penetration

From the level of the nostrils right down to the lung alveoli, the horse's respiratory system is provided with mechanical safeguards as we have seen. The construction of the nasal passages is such as to give wide surface attention to contaminants of inhaled air.

Particles larger in size than 15 microns (nm) are deposited within the nasal mucosa. From 5nm to 10nm, they can reach the trachea and bronchioles, where they are trapped in the mucociliary blanket. Particles smaller than 5nm are able to reach the lungs, where they may infect local or marauding defensive cells.

Droplet size and lung penetration can be measured in microns, as:

From 15nm to 25nm   - deposited in the upper tract
From 10nm to 20nm   - deposited in the bronchi
From 5nm to 15nm   - deposited in the bronchioles
From 2nm to 7nm   - deposited in the alveolar ducts

Particles of less than 3nm are deposited in mucus. If they get to the alveoli they are ingested by macrophages. Some are carried to lymph nodes from which they may reach the blood. Massive amounts of dirt lead to blockade of these processes and increase the chances of infection.

Factors Influencing Defence

It is important to know that the defences of the respiratory system can be interfered with by many different conditions, objects and events. Where interference does occur, the system is more likely to be invaded by organisms, especially viruses, carried in with inspired air. The causes of this interference are listed below.

1)   Chemical irritation.
2)   Mechanical suffocation.
3)   Heat, cold, and humidity.
4)   Viral effects.
5)   Nutrition and age.
6)   Stress.

We will look more closely at each of these causes in the following pages.

Chemical Irritation

Chemicals with irritant properties can damage delicate membranes when inhaled into the respiratory system and so prevent intake of oxygen. For example, ammonia, present in urine, is such an irritant and can encourage infection if allowed to build up in bedding.

As a case in point, I recall a yard of twenty suckling foals all of which had raised temperatures, increased breathing rates and ominous signs of bronchopneumonia developing in the lungs. From a clinical viewpoint, it was a worrying dilemma, with concerns over antibiotic choice and the prospect of chronically infected foals.

Because this happened on a Sunday, stable beds had only been dressed over and the tops renewed, but still there was a strong smell of ammonia. It was considered that this, coupled with the presence of a virus, was the trigger for temperature increases and infection. In the event, the boxes were properly mucked out and, within two hours, temperatures had returned to normal and breathing rates settled down - without any drugs being used. While the virus was not likely to be cleared from the system, the balance between health and infection was restored because of the removal of an irritant. No pneumonia ensued and a great deal of trouble was averted by simple management.

Mechanical Suffocation

It is quite common for mechanical suffocation to occur (for example, with inhalation of dense quantities of dust or dirt). While the respiratory system is capable of dealing with amounts of inhaled dirt, there is a limit beyond which it cannot cope. In such cases the tissues are choked and no air can reach the alveoli. Unless the situation is quickly reversed, the animal will die. Thankfully, however, this does not commonly happen.

Varying degrees of suffocation may occur, placing a burden on the health of the whole system. Macrophage activity can be affected and organisms can therefore infect more easily.

While it is easy to overstress their significance in everyday horse management, hygiene and air cleanliness are nonetheless extremely important, although healthy horses will tolerate some dust in their environment without hindrance.

A healthy, efficient respiratory system will cope with most normal challenges it is exposed to. An unhealthy, non-working system has very little chance from the start.

Heat, Cold, and Humidity

The influence of heat, cold, and humidity is very apparent when treating clinical respiratory disease in the horse. While no scientific work that establishes this statement has yet been published, it is nonetheless a fact that experiments using respiratory tissues of other animals have shown that surface chilling, excessive humidity, or heat, all have harmful effects on defensive mechanisms, including mucociliary clearance and cellular responses.

This, circumstantially, supports the contention that stabled horses have requirements for basic minimal temperatures in line with what was recommended by our forebears.

As long ago as 1869, in his book *Horses and Stables,* Lieutenant-General Sir F. Fitzwygram, Bt., wrote: 'Whilst purity of air in a stable is absolutely essential, the maintenance of an even and moderately warm temperature is also a matter of great importance.' Fitzwygram suggests that the temperature range 'be maintained between 50 and 60 degrees Fahrenheit'.

One year earlier, in 1868, W. J. Miles, MRCVSL, in his book *Modern Practical Farriery,* stated that the minimum stable temperature for a horse 'should not be less than 50 degrees Fahrenheit'.

Although today we have a completely different view being propagated in equine medicine, no scientific work has yet been done to support the change in attitudes. Many horses are subjected to wide temperature ranges while stabled - temperatures which perhaps vary more than the horses would experience outdoors. Infection appears to be a common result.

It is true that Thoroughbred horses are warm-blooded animals originating from tropical countries. Their skins are thinner and their coats lighter than that of native breeds. Many respond to heat and cold in a similar way to humans subjected to the same conditions.

Further support for this view comes from dealing with Thoroughbred foals suffering from pneumonia, where the provision of adequate heat is a critical part of treatment. In fact, it is often pointless using drugs in such cases unless the foal can be kept in a non-varying, warm environment. When this is provided, the disease is more easily treated and foals recover with fewer complications. When it is not provided, death, or chronic infection, is the frequent consequence.

In this observation, there is a direct correlation with the adult horse in training. While the older animal will much less frequently suffer from pneumonia, the incidence of low-grade respiratory infection - especially in racing age horses - is very high. It is often the provision of improper stabling that encourages this to happen, and, arguably, the consequence is the growing pool of infectious organisms that are now being isolated during disease investigations. Furthermore, many of these organisms are inconsistent in their disease producing capacity, begging the question of why this should be.

It is not unrealistic to suggest that inappropriate management - and especially where stabling is concerned - is one of the prime contributors to lowered resistance to disease and, therefore, increased virulence of organisms.

Viral Effects

Any virus infection leaves an animal weakened defensively and at a greater risk from other infections to which it may be exposed. It is possible for different viruses to infect one after another, and it is not unheard of for more than one disease causing organism to be isolated from a single disease outbreak.

A case in point is influenza which severely damages respiratory membranes and leaves animals at the mercy of secondary organisms until they are fully recovered, which may be for as long as several weeks.

Nutrition and Age

Nutritional deficiences can lead to weakness of cell structures and so influence defences. Such weakness can occur through direct deficiencies in the diet, but may also result from faulty absorbtion, improper feeding and worms.

It is also recognised that age has an adverse influence on disease susceptibility. However, this is not a major factor in dealing with infection in competing animals. Where there is increased incidence, as with chronic lung disease, the problem is often not so much an expression of lowered defensive capacity as persistent exposure to unsuitable, or intolerable, conditions.

Stress

Stress is an increasingly well recognised factor in disease - for example, it has been shown that transport and overcrowding can cause it. Scientifically, this is attributed to the influence of steroids released under stress and the advantage these give to infection.

Severe training is also stressful, as are the effects of a hard race.

Infectious disease is not the natural expression of cause and effect, of, simply, an infectious organism coming into contact with a susceptible host. If disease results it will depend on all the factors outlined in this chapter, not just of host susceptibility and resistance but also the ability of an organism to set up disease.

When it is common for low-grade, non-infectious organisms to be isolated in disease investigations, as regularly occurs, it is only natural to look for explanations. The answers are, very often, plain and simple, and may signify mistakes that have been made.

It is simple to set up infection by keeping horses in specific conditions which they cannot tolerate. For example, there are types of stables from which it is virtually impossible to produce healthy horses to race; but change to more ideal conditions and infection disappears, spontaneously, without drugs.

This is a fact that needs to be recognised and learned from.

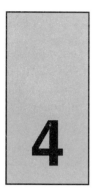

4 The Respiratory System in Disease

Diseases of the respiratory system are infectious or non-infectious. They may be categorised as follows:

Infectious
- caused by bacteria
- caused by viruses

Non-infectious
- allergic conditions
- mechanical diseases of the upper tract
- bleeding from the upper or lower tract.

We shall deal with each of these categories individually, but first we will consider some general principles relating to infection.

General Principles in Infection

In any infection the tissues of the tract are invaded by organisms, either viral or bacterial. This results initially in destruction of surface epithelial cells. The next stage sees an accumulation of serous and mucous exudates with consequent blockage of airways and reduced oxygen intake. Lung tissue may be invaded with collapse of whole areas and consolidation. Finally, the process may involve the pleura, causing pleuritis, or pleurisy, which may result in very painful breathing and adhesions forming between the lung and chest wall.

The clinical manifestations of these processes begin with increased breathing rate, temperature, pain, depression and varying degrees of nasal

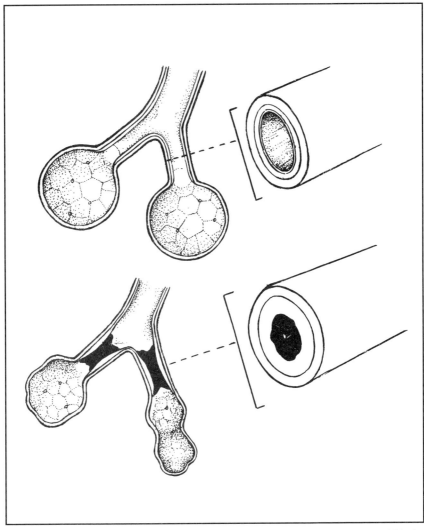

Open alveolar duct (top) *and* (bottom) *closed ducts. The latter is caused by the presence of mucus, pus, foreign matter, etc., leading to air failing to enter the alveolus which collapses*

discharge. Coughing may occur if nervous receptors are exposed and irritated. The level of temperature is variable, and its duration will depend on the organism involved (more transient with viruses, often higher and persistent with some bacterial infections). In pleurisy the affected animal may stand with its elbows abducted (held out from the body) and head extended in an effort to breathe.

Viral infections tend to be less damaging, relatively, sometimes restricting their effect to lining membranes and not achieving systemic spread to other organs through the bloodstream (viraemia). (Particular viruses, such as EHV-1, are found in the blood.) Bacterial infections, on the other hand, tend to invade tissues which have already been weakened by any of the following:

1)   Prior virus infection.
2)   Mechanical damage from irritants.
3)   Surface cell injury by toxic inhalation - of poisons or smoke.

Bacteria also have a more profound effect on the animal generally and may cause systemic spread (septicaemia). Death is more likely to ensue from a bacterial septicaemia than from viraemia. However, these are generalisations and not necessarily always the case.

Infectious Conditions Caused by Bacteria

Bacteria have been established on the planet for as long as life itself has existed. They are single cell organisms which reproduce by simple division, and are widely distributed in nature. Bacteria are readily seen under a microscope at magnifications of 1,000 times their size. They grow with ease in decomposed animal or human matter. There are varieties which live in soil; others which are vital to natural processes such as digestion; some which inhabit the surfaces of the body. Not all bacteria are harmful.

In relation to disease, there are bacteria that need oxygen for growth and others that thrive best in areas devoid of it - dead and decaying tissues are examples. Many bacteria, though not primary causes of disease, are able to set up infection if in contact with tissues which have already been debilitated.

Infection

Infection is an invasion of tissues which are then used as a basis for further growth and multiplication by the organism. Septicaemia, invasion of the bloodstream, is a serious consequence of this; it may occur as an extension from the bowel or respiratory system, or even from infected wounds.

Bacteria vary greatly in their ability to introduce disease, though their mere presence does not necessarily mean infection will occur. As we have seen, there is first a battle with body defences and the organism may well be defeated. The outcome depends on the resistance of the host, tissue damage, location of the organism in the body, and virulence.

Contagious Infection

'Contagious' means that an organism will spread rapidly; 'infectious' means it will inevitably introduce infection when it enters the body. If a disease finds an easy path from one animal to another, a contagious infection will almost certainly be present. For example, strangles is passed on by means of discharges from infected horses. If these discharges get onto a field, all other horses which subsequently graze that field may pick up the infection.

The contact can be made also through human agencies. The infection can be carried on hands and clothing, transported on buckets and other implements, food and muck sacks, etc. Remembering this is critical to control.

Spread of contagious bacterial disease

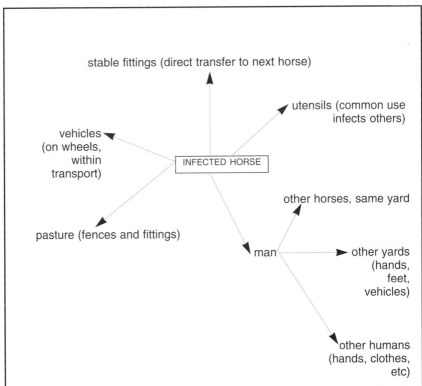

The need for control is demonstrated when anthrax is diagnosed. Anthrax is a highly infectious condition. It is spread from contaminated sources (for example, improperly sterilised meat and bone meal) and is also present in soil. Animals found to have died from this highly lethal disease are buried on the spot, under conditions which give the infection no chance to spread further.

Although anthrax is lethal it is relatively uncommon in horses; alas, strangles is not, though it kills relatively few. Anthrax is said to have a high mortality (most affected animals die) but low morbidity (few become affected). Strangles is the opposite.

Once inside the body, organisms are in a position to set up infection if the opportunity arises. If resistance is lowered (for example, through poor nutrition, management mistakes, etc.), infection is the natural sequel. And removing one organism - by antibiotic treatment - may only give opportunity to other organisms if underlying problems are not resolved.

Pneumonia

The term 'pneumonia' usually describes bacterial infection of the lungs. This may be a primary infection (in foals), or secondary to viruses and other causes (even in adults). Viral pneumonia is generally not as damaging to lung tissues as is bacterial pneumonia. However, it opens the door to bacterial infections which are more capable of causing the death of an animal.

Bronchopneumonia describes infection of the bronchi as well as lung tissue.

Where there is extensive damage to surface tissues, as in equine influenza, antibacterial defences are weakened, or wiped out, at the earliest stages of disease. In these cases there is reduced mucociliary clearance as well as lowered macrophage activity. There is also a recognised tendency for bacteria to proliferate and colonise damaged tissues. Loss of surfactant may cause the collapse of lung tissue and further inhibit cell responses because of lack of oxygen.

Any problem which lowers resistance may lead to pneumonia. Thus a combination of exposure, poor feeding and bad stabling may be the cause. It may occur when food goes the wrong way, or after worm infestations where there has been migration of larvae through the lungs.

Although specific organisms, such as *Streptococci* and *Pasteurella* species, are commonly associated with equine pneumonia it is debatable as to whether primary bacterial pneumonia occurs in the adult animal.

Generally the disease is seen in isolated cases and is not contagious. Where there is an exception to this, some scientific opinion believes that it is usually due to an underlying problem affecting resistance. Also, if the infection is allowed to spread, the organism may gain virulence and become more infectious.

Symptoms

A significant rise of temperature occurs at an early stage, accompanied by an increase in respiratory rate and pulse. The animal may sweat slightly or be seen to shiver. There may or may not be a cough, and nasal discharges may occur but are not consistently seen. The nostrils are dilated and if there is associated pleurisy - which is an extension of the infection onto the linings of the chest cavity - there is marked pain on breathing.

Depending on the organism involved and the length of time the infection has existed, abscesses can occur. This is especially common in *Rhodococcus equi* infection of foals. The presence of abscesses makes the condition more difficult to treat and considerably extends the period of recovery.

In some apparently healthy horses, areas of pneumonia can be detected in the lungs on auscultation (listening) with a stethoscope, without the presence of temperature change or other external signs, except perhaps for reduced exercise tolerance and mild changes in respiration at rest. When examined by endoscope, no abnormality may be detected. Such horses may suffer acute respiratory distress after a gallop and may make gurgling sounds during the course of a race. They tend, however, to respond well to treatment.

Diagnosis

Parts of the lung are attacked and become consolidated with no entry of air into them. These areas can be detected with the help of a stethoscope and neighbouring areas usually are marked by abnormal sounds caused by exudates in the air passages. The symptoms, generally, are very typical and the condition is easily diagnosed on seeing them.

Diagnosis can be confirmed by radiography, various forms of thermal imaging and diagnostic ultrasound.

Treatment

Antibiotics are indicated early, and the response is likely to be good. The horse must be kept warm and out of draughts. The atmosphere must be clean and healthy so that oxygen is readily available - as there is reduced lung space for gas exchange. However, it is dangerous to allow stable temperatures to fall in the process of providing air, so both requirements have to be met within reason.

Many horses will not recover from this condition while kept in sub-optimal conditions - though will respond spontaneously when the right conditions are provided.

The prognosis with pneumonia today is good. The animal will need professional attendance, but may make a complete recovery in a matter of days in response to effective treatment.

The use of bronchodilators and mucous clearing drugs in this condition is often disappointing. However, the management of the animal is critical to recovery and full return to normal occurs through judicious care.

Pleurisy

('Pleuritis' is the more correct term, though pleurisy is commonly used in medical circles). Pleurisy is an inflammation of the pleura, the covering membrane of the lungs and chest cavity. It normally occurs as an extension of infection from the lung itself or, rarely, as a consequence of penetrating wounds of the chest wall.

Symptoms

This is a painful condition that causes discomfort while breathing. There is an increased respiratory rate with quick, shallow breaths, raised temperature, and quite frequently the animal is reluctant to move. In the early stages, a horse might be bright but off food and displaying evident signs of pain.

As the condition progresses the symptoms become more exaggerated until the animal exhibits severe respiratory embarrassment. Accumulation of fluid exudate in the chest cavity may further inhibit gas transfer in the lungs by causing collapse of dependent areas. Adhesions may also form between the lung and chest wall, further complicating the condition.

Diagnosis

Pleurisy is diagnosed on the basis of the symptoms and it is important that this be done early before fluid accumulates and respiration becomes more

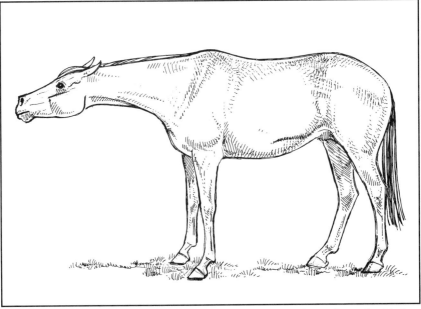

A horse suffering from pleurisy will experience acute pain and stand with legs apart, head extended and nostrils flared

difficult. Auscultation is characteristic with typical sounds created by friction between the inflamed membranes.Radiography will reveal the extent of fluid accumulations in advanced cases.

Treatment

Prompt intravenous treatment with effective antibiotics will very often resolve the condition without further complication. More chronic cases may require aspiration of accumulated fluid and recovery may be prolonged.

It is vital that horses suffering from this condition be kept warm and out of draughts but with adequate oxygen supply and good nourishing food.

Infectious Conditions Caused by Viruses

Because of their smaller size, the historical identification of viruses was more recent - although we now know that particular virus families have existed throughout recorded time. As a practical recognition of this, the Chinese are known to have infected their children with smallpox from established adult skin lesions as early as the eleventh century. Human influenza virus was first isolated in 1933 in the United Kingdom, while the equine equivalent was not identified until 1956 in Prague. Yet history records the depredations of a flu-like infection in horse populations going back hundreds of years.

The most noteworthy ways in which viruses differ from bacteria are their much smaller size and their manner of life. Viruses are measured in millimicrons - a micron being a millionth of a metre; a millimicron is a thousand times smaller than a micron. Viruses are not complete in themselves; they cannot live and reproduce except in the substance of living cells. They do not survive for long in nature.

Outside the body, viruses are subject to death from drying, heat, chemicals, exposure to the sun, etc. However, they may live for a limited time in discharges which protect them from these hazards and they are preserved to a degree by freezing (contrary to common belief). Viruses are obliged to get back into living tissue in order to grow, multiply and spread. Outside living tissue, viruses are not dead, but inert, and their chances of survival are reduced. They thrive on perpetuating disease, so ensuring their own continuance. They must spread internally to produce infection and be shed into the environment to perpetuate their species.

Viruses also have to face the same defensive systems as bacteria. Their great advantage is their small size, which allows easy penetration to deeper lung tissues in air - their most common vehicle of entry into the body. They also have the ability to grow rapidly, and to constantly produce new varieties - by a process called mutation.

On the other hand, viruses, while often tending to be very contagious are not always highly infectious. In many cases their ability to introduce disease is dependent on a lowering of the resistance of the host. The most common cycle of infection with respiratory viruses is short - a matter of days - but this is extended by the host's weakness or any external factor that contributes to it.

The spread of viruses is much the same as for bacteria (generally contained in discharges which may be picked up by hands, clothing, etc.) but with one major difference. The most important source of spread in the United Kingdom and Ireland is in air contaminated with infected respiratory discharges. In other countries (for example, the USA, Africa, Spain) biting flies are commonly involved in the spread of certain viruses (arboviruses) and there is evidence that some species of bird can act as reservoir hosts for viruses such as influenza. It is suspected that these hosts may well play a part in the production of new virus strains found in horses.

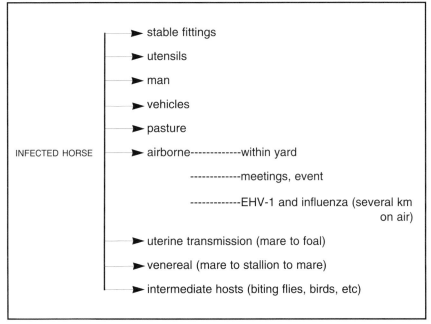

INFECTED HORSE
- ► stable fittings
- ► utensils
- ► man
- ► vehicles
- ► pasture
- ► airborne-------------within yard

  -------------meetings, event

  -------------EHV-1 and influenza (several km on air)
- ► uterine transmission (mare to foal)
- ► venereal (mare to stallion to mare)
- ► intermediate hosts (biting flies, birds, etc)

Spread of virus disease

When coughed or blown out of the nasal passages, viruses will travel for varying distances depending on particle size. The influenza virus is directly coughed into the air and so reaches other horses in an immediate building, or at a sales yard, a race meeting or event. Yet, in one outbreak in South Africa, influenza virus was reported to have travelled several kilometres by air (in the United Kingdom it was previously thought that the virus was borne by air over only short distances). The herpes virus, EHV-1, the cause of abortion in mares, is known to travel long distances on the wind (put at 30km or more and certainly appearing to do so in clinical situations). This is a major factor in the spread of this disease. Horses cough little with herpesvirus infection, but they do clear their noses in an explosive way that has a similar effect.

In clinical EHV-1 outbreaks it has been known for horses in fields close to animals suffering abortion and paralysis to be free of these symptoms. What this means in a clinical context is not wholly clear. However, the outdoor (abortion and paralysis free) animals usually show gross clinical signs of the virus (marked by nasal discharges, discoloured membranes, etc.) and it is probable that the effect of congregation of animals within stable units is a critical factor in the development of this disease. It also means that diluting infection by turning horses out can play a vital part in control in almost any virulent virus outbreak.

Virulence and Mutation

Virulence is a measure of an organism's ability to enter animal tissues and set up infection. In virus infection, particularly, virulence increases as an infection builds up and passes from animal to animal. Along with mutation, which allows for the development of viral variation, virulence has a significant influence on the spread of disease.

Mutation is a feature of all viral infections; it contributes to virulence because it helps to sidestep body defences.

Viral Pneumonia

Pneumonia of purely viral origin (also called pneumonitis) - that is, not complicated by bacteria - is marked by loss of epithelial cells and mobilisation of white blood cells, particularly neutrophils and lymphocytes. As a direct result of this, exudates gather in the alveoli and prevent access of air to the respiratory surfaces. Furthermore, the destruction of tissues opens the path to secondary invaders, including bacteria.

In healthy animals, there is an immediate assault on invading viruses, many of which are consumed and killed off at an early stage. Progress of the infection depends on the virulence of the virus, the quantity of the challenge (the physical amount of virus involved) and the immune status of the host animal.

Mucociliary clearance is a vital aspect of respiratory defences, but deeper lung areas lack ciliated cells and depend on macrophages to trap organisms and other foreign matter. In infection, this effort is helped by the influx of other white blood cells and antibodies. Anything that inhibits macrophage activity would aid viral infection. Although there is a lack of evidence to establish that this happens in existing disease patterns, it is a considered possibility.

Symptoms

There may be temperature increases, increase in respiration, mild watery discharge from the nostrils. However, without secondary bacterial involvement, the symptoms may be so mild as to go unnoticed in older animals. In young foals, the effect of viruses such as EHV-1 often cause severe illness soon after birth with symptoms of pneumonia and death at an early stage. If these animals have become infected in the womb there is little chance they will survive.

Post-natal infections of Arab foals suffering from immune deficiency with adenovirus is often fatal.

Treatment

There is little in the way of drug treatment that is effective against virus infections.

However, foals born healthy have a good chance of fighting common infections if they get adequate colostrum from their dams.

Older horses will normally recover if given rest, warmth and are adequately nourished.

Infection of the Newborn

Respiratory stress in a newborn foal is often an indication of prematurity and reflects collapse of lung tissues due to a failure of development of surfactant. Such stress can also occur as an expression of prenatal infection with organisms such as EHV-1.

In foals of a few days old, primary pneumonia is uncommon although lung infection due to septicaemic spread is not. Many such conditions are caused by post-natal, or perinatal, infection and are very closely linked with the effectiveness of immune transfer from the dam.

Pneumonia in any foal, because of problems of immunity, is always more difficult to treat than in the adult animal. The provision of absolute external temperature stability is a critical part of treatment.

Localised Diseases of Infectious Origin

These are numerous and here we can describe only some of those which are most often encountered.

Sinusitis

Infection of the horse's sinuses occurs either as an extension from disease of the upper respiratory tract or as a sequel to tooth infection; it can involve any individual sinus.

Symptoms

A unilateral purulent discharge is common when the infection is patent, or open (pus is able to drain from the infected sinuses, seen at the nostril). There is often pain on percussion (gentle tapping with a finger) over the area. If the infection is closed, the sinus fills with pus and the bone may become deformed, with evident distortion of the outline of the face. The eye may water on the affected side.

Diagnosis

Endosopic examination will locate the source of a discharge, radiography will help to locate an infection and define the sinuses affected. If the infection has been caused by a tooth, this may also be detected on radiograph.

Treatment

Antibiotics may be effective in open cases. Where drainage is not occurring, surgery is performed under general anaesthesia and the sinus is entered by means of a trephine (a surgical instrument to penetrate bone) and the infection is allowed to drain externally. The sinus will continue to be flushed daily until the infection has been overcome. If an abnormal tooth is found to be the cause of the problem, this may be removed at the same time.

Pharyngeal Lymphoid Hyperplasia

The condition known as pharyngeal lymphoid hyperplasia (PLH) has received greater attention since the advent of the fibreoptic endoscope.

Some authorities consider PLH to be of little clinical significance, though others associate it with current infection and advise antibiotic treatment.

PLH is marked by inflammatory changes in the lymphoid tissue of the pharyngeal region, including on the soft palate, epiglottis and within the gutteral pouches. These vary from small white spots to large polyps which intrude on the airway and are capable of causing abnormal noises during respiration.

The condition occurs after bacterial and viral infections, also after the inhalation of irritants and allergens. The incidence of PLH is high in young horses and gradually decreases as they get older. Some horses suffer from the condition throughout their two-year-old and three-year-old racing careers, but the relationship with performance is disputed as many animals with PLH perform up to expectations.

It must also be considered that PLH is a response to ongoing external stress, such as faulty environment or poor stabling.

Gutteral Pouch Disease

Empyema (build up of pus) of the gutteral pouch is a purulent infection, often as an extension from infected glands in the region. There may be swelling of the pouch, nasal discharge, pain in the area and difficulty with swallowing and breathing. Surgery may be required if the condition fails to respond to antibiotic therapy.

Gutteral pouch mycosis is a fungal infection which occurs mainly in stabled horses. The condition can be without symptoms, or there can be sporadic bleeding episodes while the horse is at rest if the infection has managed to damage blood vessels in the region. The bleeding is usually confined to one nostril, but may be bilateral.

Damage to nerves as a result of gutteral pouch problems can cause paralysis of the pharynx and the return of food through the nostrils.

Tympany (ballooning) of the gutteral pouch is mentioned here for convenience though it is not an infectious condition. It is occasionally seen in young horses, the pouch being ballooned by air. It is marked by varying degrees of swelling in the region below the ear and is usually painless. Tympany may resolve itself spontaneously or can be relieved by surgery.

Diagnosis

Specific diagnosis requires endoscopy, which helps to identify the source of the bleeding, or discharge, to the gutteral pouch opening into the pharynx. Bleeding could alternatively arise from the ethmoid area at the back of the nasal passages or from fracture of the hyoid bone, which may injure blood vessels in the gutteral pouch area.

Treatment

It is possible to treat gutteral pouch mycosis using modern antifungal drugs which can be instilled straight into the affected pouch. Where the lesion is extensive and serious damage occurs to one of the major blood vessels surgery may be an option. However, in some cases, the haemorrhage cannot be stemmed and the condition proves fatal.

Allergic Conditions

Allergic conditions of the respiratory tract are most commonly caused by bacterial and fungal spores, pollens and dust (all called allergens) which are inhaled from hay, straw and other bedding. Tissues become sensitised when they meet an allergen and then respond to renewed contact by becoming inflamed. This may cause the narrowing of airways to the lungs. The above allergens may contaminate the environment of a building and be blown into the atmosphere from fittings and recesses even by animals coughing.

Mechanical Diseases of the Upper Tract

Mechanical diseases of the horse's respiratory tract include laryngeal hemiplegia (ILH), although conditions such as dorsal displacement of the soft palate (DDSP) are equally important. All such conditions, explained in greater detail later, are relevant to reasons under which horses could be, and are, rejected after sale. For example, in the United States, sales catalogues expressly mention the following conditions, in identical terms:
1)   Laryngeal hemiplegia.
2)   Rostral displacement of the palatopharyngeal arch.
3)   Epiglottic entrapment.
4   Permanent dorsal displacement of the soft palate.
5)   Severe arytenoid chondritis or chondroma.
6)   Subepiglottic cyst.

Bleeding from the Upper or Lower Tract

Bleeding can occur from any part of the respiratory tract; however, it is most common in particular areas. Thus, bleeding at rest may emanate from the gutteral pouches or from growths in the nasal passages or over the ethmoid area. Bleeding during racing is most commonly localised to dorsal areas of the lungs.

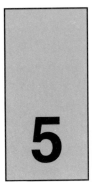

5 Infectious Disease Investigation

Epidemiology is the discipline of disease investigation. It involves the isolation and identification of the underlying causes of disease, as well as defining where and when it occurs, how many animals are affected and how a condition is spread. Its conclusions aim at an understanding of how infection might be controlled, as well as assessing how such control measures might work.

This chapter considers the laboratory aspects of the process.

Samples

Infectious material sent for laboratory examination is normally contained in suitable transport media. Viral samples may contain antibiotics to stem bacterial growth or contain additives to stabilise contained viruses. These are transported (packed in ice) at a temperature ranging from freezing to 4 degrees C. For bacterial isolation, swabs are also transported in media which help to foster survival of the organism until it can be cultured. However, bacteria are easier to grow on artificial media and simpler to identify because of their larger size.

Swabs, Washes and Scrapings

Nasal and pharyngeal swabs, tracheal washes, scrapings, and biopsies are taken for culture and electronmicroscopy to identify viral particles and the presence of defensive tissue reactions.

These are all aids in the diagnosis of disease and play an important part in identifying the cause.

Culturing Bacteria

At the laboratory, a swab from an infected site is smeared onto a plate of sterile culture material, like blood agar, and placed in an incubator. Within twenty-four hours, a growth will appear in most positive cases. The organism can then be identified by various tests and by its appearance when examined under a microscope. A sensitivity test can be carried out to discover what antibiotics will be most effective against it. This is done by laying a fresh growth onto another plate containing numerous small discs of different antibiotics. The bacteria will gradually invade the areas around those discs to which they are resistant. Clear areas with no growth indicate that an organism is vulnerable to antibiotics in the related discs. The animal is then treated on the basis of this information.

In acute conditions it is not possible to wait for test results, so treatment has to be started immediately. However, a sensitivity result may be available if further treatment is needed and this can be of benefit.

It is important that any bacterial infection is terminated as soon as is possible in order to limit damage to tissues, yet there are many situations

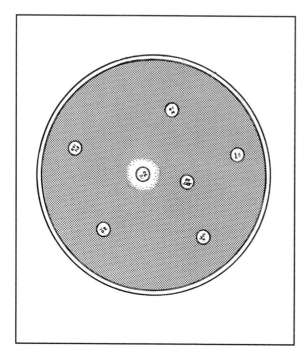

Schematic drawing of a blood-agar plate on which a sensitivity test is being carried out. The white discs are impregnated with antibiotic. A clear area around a disc indicates the organism being cultured is susceptible to the specific antibiotic in the disc

in which it is not easy to take a swab. Then the treating veterinary surgeon has to rely on knowledge and instinct to reach a cure.

Isolation and Identification of Viruses

Virus isolation is considerably more difficult than is the culturing of bacteria; it is also, generally, a great deal slower, being achieved by growth on laboratory media that include living tissue and embryonated eggs.

Isolation depends on a sick animal being in an infectious condition (actually shedding virus) at the time samples are taken, also that the virus in question is one that will grow under laboratory conditions. When it is understood that the infectious state only persists for a limited time, it can be accepted that negative results mean very little. And, it must be added, the isolation of a virus (or bacterium) does not necessarily mean it is the cause of the disease in question.

The electron microscope has made it possible to recognise and identify individual viruses, by magnifying their size by up to half a million times. This has allowed them to be put into separate categories and classified by family.

Blood Analysis

Blood analysis plays a part in modern infectious disease management, even though its effectiveness is open to criticism. It is divided into three distinct categories: haematology; biochemistry; and serology.

Haematology is the examination of the cellular elements of the blood, while biochemistry is analysis of the chemical elements; serology is the testing for antibodies.

Blood analysis involves routine examination for significant changes that might indicate disease. The changes are:
1)   Alteration of the white cell content.
2)   Alteration of circulating fluid volume.
3)   Interference with oxygen carrying capacity.
4)   Enzyme responses to tissue destruction.
5)   Imbalance or deficiency of minerals and trace elements.

It should be appreciated from the outset that both haematology and biochemistry are essentially aids to diagnosis, and not a diagnostic element in themselves.

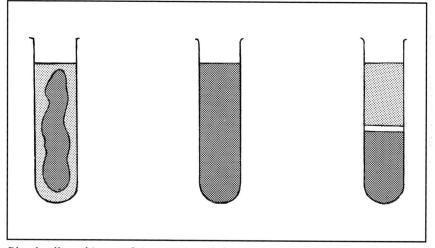

Blood collected into a plain container (left) *will clot; blood remains whole when collected into a container* (centre) *that contains an anticoagulant; whole blood* (right), *when left standing, will separate. The separation being: into red blood cells (which fall to the bottom), white blood cells (which sit on top of the red blood cells) and a clear plasma layer*

This means that, in addition to blood analysis, a clinical examination must be conducted to gauge the influence of minor changes in blood pictures. It also suggests that the interpretations of tests by laboratories are notoriously fallible.

Information from this source, as presently available, is often, at best, only scratching the surface of disease interpretation. Positive results can occur in situations where disease influences are negligible. Negative results may be associated with horses suffering from severe illness that should not be worked or raced. In fact, without competent clinical opinion, these tests are frequently not worth their cost.

Haematology

In dealing with horses in training, haematology is used to help establish the presence or absence of infection, and it is only fair to say that results are open to error. It should be understood that haematology does not identify specific infectious diseases.

The kind of viral infections involved are often negligible in clinical effect and generally not noticed in horses which are not competing. On the other hand, they have a profound effect on immediate ability to perform

HAEMATOLOGY	normal ranges (SI units)
Total red blood cells	6-12
Haemoglobin	11-16
Haematocrit (packed cell volume)	0.33-0.49
MCV (mean corpuscular volume)	36-49
MCHC (mean corpuscular haemoglobin concentration)	29-36
Total white blood cells	4-11
Neutrophils	2-7 (about 60%)*
Lymphocytes	1-6 (about 40%)*
Monocytes	0-0.4
Eosinophils	0-0.3
Basophils	0-0.1

BIOCHEMISTRY	normal ranges	
Total protein	60-80	g/l
Albumin	27-40	g/l
Globulin	17-34	g/l
Plasma viscosity (PV)	1.40-1.70	centipoises
Plasma fibrinogen	0-3.0	g/l
Serum amyloid	0-200	u/l
Alkaline phosphatase	0-145	u/l
Bilirubin	10-40	mmol/l
Urea	3.5-7.3	mmol/l
AST/SGOT	0-250	u/l
CK/CPK	0-100	mmol/l
Calcium (Ca)	2.6-3.9	mmol/l
Phosphorus (P)	0.8-1.8	mmol/l
Ca:P ratio	3:1	

*Expressed as a percentage of total white blood cell count

A typical blood profile showing normal range limits

and are probably the most common cause of performance problems encountered in racehorses.

The variation in cellular blood levels in these cases is very often marginal and difficult to interpret. It may not be possible to tell if a horse is actively infected by, recovering from, or simply incubating disease. Bacterial infections have a more marked influence especially on white blood cells, and are more debilitating - and easier to diagnose clinically.

The initial response to a viral infection is often a mild relative dehydration, with increased total red blood cell count, packed cell volume (also called PCV or haematocrit) and depression of white blood cell numbers. This response is often followed by a drop in red blood cell numbers and packed cell volume. There are, too, changes to the white blood cell count depending on the organism and the effect it has.

However, it is commonly found that haematology does not parallel the specific clinical condition and that results indicate normality rather than disease (described as 'within normal limits') when the animal clearly is not normal.

The opposite also is found, where an abnormal result emerges although the animal has already recovered. The breadth of normal ranges is often too wide in practice, and horses will sometimes perform well at either extreme of these, while only the smallest variation can be significant in some cases.

In using haematology for disease control the above limitations have got to be considered.

The following items are routinely tested for in haematology, and are measured in standard SI (Système International d'Unités) units.

Red Blood Cells
A normal range of 6 to 12 units per litre. At either end of this range it is likely that performance would suffer although an animal still might not be clinically ill.

Haemoglobin
Range varies from 11 to 16 units per litre. For a racehorse in training the optimal level is close to 14.

Packed Cell Volume (PCV)
Range varies from 0.33 to 0.49 units. The lower of these levels is normal for horses engaged in long-distance work but not for racing animals (although some racehorses defy low packed cell volume levels if allowed to conserve energy, as long as there is no underlying disease). The higher level would very probably limit performance because of dehydration. Levels between 0.40 and 0.42 are generally acceptable in racing animals except where they signify a sudden change from an animal's normal level.

Mean Corpuscular Volume (MCV)
A further guide to the oxygen carrying capacity of the blood.

Mean Corpuscular Haemoglobin Concentration (MCHC)
Another guide to the oxygen carrying capacity of the blood.

White Blood Cells
Range varies from 4 to 11 units per litre of blood. The lower end of the range could signify the early stages of virus infection while the higher might well be associated with significant, localised bacterial activity.

Neutrophils
White cells which respond to bacterial infection, neutrophils are measured at a normal unit range of 2 to 7 per litre. The percentage of neutrophils against total white blood cells is also usually measured at about 60 per cent

Lymphocytes
Lymphocytes are closely associated with immune responses to infection and can appear in chronic bacterial as well as viral conditions. Range varies from 1 to 6 units per litre and lymphocytes normally constitute about 40 per cent of white blood cells.

Monocytes
In some viral conditions monocytes will be present. The range varies from 0 to 0.4 units per litre.

Eosinophils
Seen in allergic and parasitic conditions. Range varies from 0 to 0.3 units per litre.

Basophils
Cells involved in immune responses, basophils contain histamine and heparin which they release into the blood in inflammatory situations. Range varies from 0 to 0.1 units per litre.

Biochemistry

The range of biochemical tests is constantly being extended and varied; scientists are continually trying to improve the quality of the information provided and to overcome present failings in the system. However, it may be that the answer to their problem is more constructive clinical opinion.

Some Routine Tests

Restrictions on space in this book does not allow a detailed description of all biochemical tests. However, the following text describes some of the more common, or everyday, tests.

Total Protein
Helpful in assessing nutritional status and the influence of parasitic or infectious disease.

Albumin and Globulin
Useful in differentiating liver conditions. Specific globulin fractions can indicate tissue damage due to worms and bacterial or viral infections.

Plasma Viscosity (PV)
A non-specific guide to inflammatory disease, used often by trainers as a screen on horses in training.

Plasma Fibrinogen
Elevated levels indicate tissue damage and may help with diagnosis of internal abscesses, chronic infection, internal parasites and pulmonary haemorrhage.

Serum Amyloid
Recently researched and promising to provide useful information in the diagnosis of septic lesions and their ongoing supervision.

Alkaline Phosphatase
Raised blood levels occur in liver disease, bowel abnormalities and some bone conditions.

Bilirubin
As an adjunct to the diagnosis of liver disease and anaemia.

Urea
Elevated levels indicate uraemia due to faulty kidney function.

Aspartate Aminotransferase (AST or SGOT)
Raised blood levels indicate muscle and/or liver damage.

Creatine Kinase (CK)
Levels raised in muscle damage.

Blood tests for muscle damage are intended for differential diagnosis (but, for example, in acute muscle injury, there are evident external signs of muscle impairment and the condition is easily diagnosed from the symptoms). After clinical virus disease, muscle dysfunction often occurs in horses at work and appears to be linked to liver damage caused by viruses such as EHV-1. It is, therefore, not a primary muscle damage (as would occur when a muscle is torn in an uninfected horse) and usually resolves itself as the effects of the infection pass off. It is often complicated by feeding excessive levels of protein in the diet at this time.

Blood level tests of minerals and trace elements are also routinely carried out. Of these, calcium, phosphorus and magnesium are especially important.

Serology

Serology is a common diagnostic tool, in which blood or serum samples taken from infected animals are tested for antibodies to identify specific viruses or bacteria. In some cases it is necessary to examine paired samples taken about two weeks apart to confirm that an active disease process exists. This is established where there is a rising blood response (i.e. the level of antibodies rises) against the virus in question.

For the direct ELISA (enzyme linked immunoabsorbent assay) test, a suspect serum sample is added to a plate containing a given virus. After a time, an enzyme labelled antibody to horse antibody is added, followed by a substrate for the enzyme. Colour change which can be measured reflects the amount of antibody to the virus present in the sample.

Other serologic procedures are used: for example, virus neutralisation, radioimmunoassay, complement fixation, single radial hemolysis, and haemagglutination inhibition. (Haemagglutination is the capacity to cause red blood cells to clump together, caused by antibodies, viruses, etc.)

In recent years a radioisotopic antiglobulin binding assay has been developed for influenza; although it does not differentiate between the two subtypes, it is sensitive and rapid.

Serology, like haematology and biochemistry, also has its drawbacks, except where a positive diagnosis can be made with speed. Horse owners do not, as a rule, appreciate the benefit of a result that takes time to produce and does not influence the progress of a disease or the treatment of an affected horse. The value of positive diagnosis, however, exists in the need to identify organisms so that disease patterns can be better understood and so facilitate control in a wider sense. With slowly spreading viruses it allows management procedures to be introduced to restrict spread.

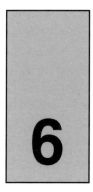

6 Diagnosis, Treatment and Management

While the diagnosis, treatment and management of respiratory disease is usually a task for the professional, there is a great deal that a horse owner can do, by observation, to detect overt changes in a horse's condition.

Diagnosis

It is important to be totally familiar with the normal processes of respiration and the external characteristics of the tract.

In this chapter we concentrate on the examination of a horse thought to be suffering from a respiratory condition. There are a number of steps to the examination which ultimately will lead to a diagnosis.

1)   Study and recognise the normal breathing rate and pattern in the horse at rest. The rate should be in the range of 8 to 12 breaths per minute, and the character of breathing should be smooth and rythmical with a long, steady intake of air and a pause between successive breaths. This pause shortens as the breathing rate increases and disappears completely at higher rates.

Faster rates at rest may occur in the absence of disease because of excitement, humidity, or reduced oxygen content of air (as would happen at altitude for example).

Even marginal changes in rate and pattern may be significant in a resting horse, so, if present, look for other signs.

2)   Be aware of the character and the depth of respiration change in disease. There is often a marked tendency to abdominal breathing and early development of a light heave-line. Double expiratory efforts indicate

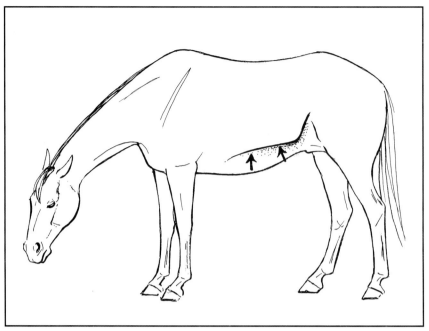

Horses suffering from chronic respiratory disease often display a heave line (arrowed) *under the belly*

that the horse's lungs are unable to empty of air (the added abdominal effort is intended to force air from lungs not automatically emptying, where elastic recoil has been lost).

Breaks in the inspiratory pattern, with flaring of the nostrils and increased effort to inhale are significant. Horses suffering severe oxygen deficiencies may stand with their elbows abducted and head and neck extended; however, extreme though this condition is, and unmistakable, it is important to be able to detect the very earliest changes for effective disease control.

3)   Check the colour of the nasal, and other, mucous membranes. While there is natural congestion after exercise, inflamed membranes at rest can indicate infection or allergy. Severely congested membranes, which may be difficult to differentiate from infected ones, are sometimes caused by heart disease. Yellowing of the membranes (jaundice) is often seen in EHV-1 infection, in which the discoloration varies from the palest yellow to more pronounced tones. More marked jaundice is seen in other conditions causing liver damage, including some forms of poisoning. Purple discoloration of the membranes is typical of rhinopneumonitis (EHV-1 and 4).

When in doubt, compare the colour of the nasal mucous membrane with that of the mouth and eye. In systemic conditions each will be equally affected.

4)   Palpate the lymph glands inside the angle of the horse's jaw. Any activity or enlargement in these glands is usually an indication of current infection.

5)   Examine the larynx carefully and form an opinion as to whether the left side is less well developed than the right side. In the presence of an abnormal inspiratory noise when exercised, this finding may have significance. Whistling and roaring are often due to paralysis affecting the left side of the larynx.

6)   Note the presence of any nasal discharges. While a slight watery discharge is normal, especially in cold weather, any evident increase is significant, especially when colour changes are detected in the membranes. Thickening of discharge may indicate bacterial infection, especially if there is pus in it.

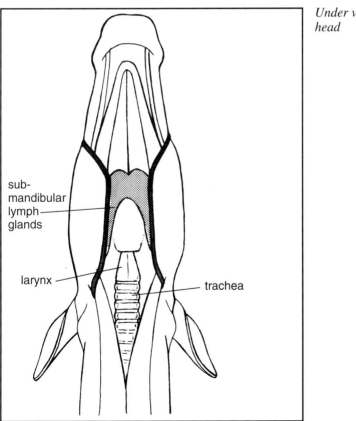

Under view of the head

sub-
mandibular
lymph
glands

larynx

trachea

Horses with chronic COPD (chronic obstructive pulmonary disease) develop a whitish discharge at exercise which is often frothy and may contain inflammatory material (detectable microscopically).

However, many horses in poor condition produce similar kinds of discharge resulting from congestion, or infection, or from being kept in stale, badly-ventilated stables. These discharges will disappear as the horses' health and physical fitness improve with training.

It is important to note if the discharge is unilateral (restricted to one nostril), or bilateral. Discharges from sinus infections are usually unilateral, thick and purulent in nature. Bilateral discharges are commonly indicative of disease in the lower tract, as in influenza.

Blood as a constituent of nasal discharge is a critical factor. Bilateral discharge of blood most often originates from the horse's lung, whereas unilateral blood is most commonly from the region of the nasal passage of the affected side, the ethmoid area at the back, or the gutteral pouch on the same side (which may also produce bilateral discharge of blood).

Food in nasal discharge can occur in some infectious conditions, such as strangles. It can also result from pharyngeal paralysis or injury to the larynx from a foreign body, such as a piece of wood.

7) If a horse is in training, any lengthening of the recovery period after exercise is significant and will need thorough investigation. The most probable cause is lung disease, though it could also result from any interference with oxygen transport, as would happen in anaemia.

It can also indicate myocarditis, a very serious problem in some virus infections.

8) Any abnormal inspiratory sounds at exercise are likely to be important in diagnosis and require professional investigation.

These steps concluded, the examination from this point on is a matter for professional opinion and may involve endoscopy, endotracheal washes for laboratory material and, conceivably, radiography or other forms of advanced lung imaging.

Endoscopy is increasingly used today, both as an aid to diagnosis, where it is extremely useful in sourcing abnormal discharges, and for the detailed examination of the nasal passages, pharynx, larynx, trachea and bronchi. By transmitting light to these internal structures a clear view can be obtained at the eyepiece and samples can also be taken for laboratory examination.

However, it should be appreciated that endoscopy has its limitations and that the absence of detectable signs of disease does not automatically mean health of the respiratory system. Nonetheless, used judiciously, endoscopy is a welcome addition to veterinary practice and enlarges the scope for wider disease identification.

Treatment

It is not possible to be too specific on the subject of treatment. All treatment must depend on correct diagnosis and each individual case will have its own requirements. But, principally, the onset of respiratory disease is very often as a result of management error; treatment therefore requires the detection and correction of such errors. Without this, drug therapy is irrational (treating the consequence, not the cause) and is only likely to create further problems.

In bacterial infections antibiotics may be indicated and these are, in ideal circumstances, prescribed on the basis of sensitivity tests (or the vet's choice for immediate use). Other drugs may also be used to relieve symptoms of congestion, to encourage the breakdown of pus and mucus and help its elimination from the tract.

Drugs may also be used to alleviate inflammation and to dilate air passages and improve ventilation of the lung. In illness, and sometimes after competing, oxygen therapy may be indicated and this may be administered with a mask or by the introduction of a tube into a single nostril.

As a preventive against COPD, drugs by inhalation may be used - and antibiotics are sometimes given by this method for resistant infections of localised areas of the tract.

Very occasionally, where there is incurable obstruction of the horse's upper respiratory tract (of the nature of ILH or DDSP) a tracheostomy is carried out. This operation involves making a permanent opening into the trachea at about the middle third of the neck and inserting a metal tube through which a horse can breathe, for example, when racing. While this operation can prove effective, it is very important, quite evidently, that no mud or dirt block the opening during the course of the race.

Management

Recognising and controlling infection is the first step in managing respiratory disease.

It is recognised that population increases opportunity for disease. Therefore, the more horses on a premises, or in a district, the greater will be the scope for organisms to establish themselves and spread. While it may appear that there is little that can be done to influence this state of affairs, no infection should ever be encouraged to run its course. To take no action leads to greater virulence and weakens resistance against other infections. In effect, to be off guard is to invite trouble.

Spread of Infection

Vigilance is needed in any equine management system and none more so than in preventing the spread of infection.

On most premises natural comings and goings leave an open channel to the outside world. Racehorses, other competition horses and broodmares may all enter and leave, bringing with them possible contact infections. Very often, these simple comings and goings pave the way for whole episodes of disease; and not necessarily always because there are too many horses, but because one or two - perhaps for avoidable reasons - are more open to infection.

There is the possibility, particularly when mares collect on stud farms, that animals coming from different locations may arrive with similar symptoms of disease. It happens regularly in virus abortion crises, and is of interest to those who deal in epidemiology.

International competition, too, creates a prospect for wider dissemina-

Spread of bacterial infection within a yard

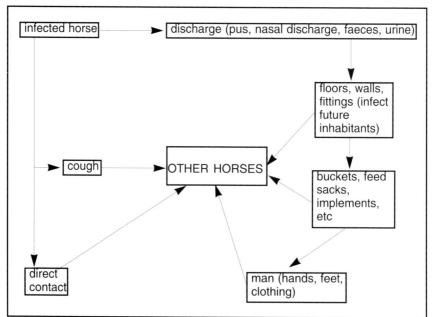

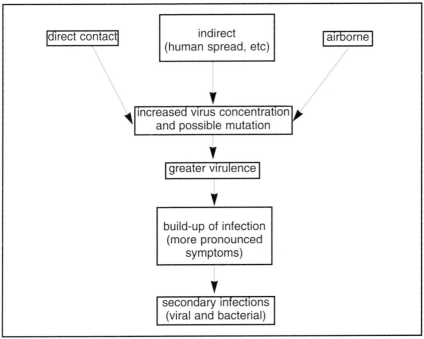

Spread of viral infection within a yard. Control therefore requires the dispersal of badly-affected animals (though this may not be allowed with some infections) to dilute the level of infection. Isolation of susceptible animals and tightening of hygiene and disinfection programmes is also recommended. Antibiotics may be used to control secondary bacterial infections

tion, sometimes of diseases which are not native and which may not be detected at the time horses are examined before departure from foreign countries. Happily, though, nature tends to place her own limitations on the movement of infection - for example, the serious outbreak of African horse sickness (AHS) in Spain in the years before the 1992 Olympic Games ventured no further north in Europe. That the transmitting vector (in the case of AHS especially) has so far not appeared to adapt to climatic change, is one important reason for optimism; and there may be other unknown reasons why infecting organisms do not become established out of their recognised territories. Yet, we are warned, if global warming becomes a reality, we may in time be confronted with a different prospect.

Control of Infection

Methods of control will vary and will also depend on resources and staff available. Some control methods are examined here.

Isolation

Though frequently used in connection with infection in horses, 'isolation' is a word which is subject to a certain amount of misunderstanding. In the context of virus infection, isolation means not only complete separation but the exclusion of all possible contamination. To be fully effective, even air would have to be filtered.

However, quite often horses respond to a partial type of isolation because the conditions under which they are kept help to overcome the infection they bear.

Preventive Medicine

In racing and most competition events, there is a clearer understanding of the need for preventive medicine as opposed to the purely curative type. Horses will not race when infected and it is far more economical to prevent problems rather than to try to treat, or live with, them.

An essential element of prevention is in good management and in the understanding of health, resistance and the nature of infectious organisms.

Infections often start by contact with outside sources - at race meetings, competitions, sales, even on communal gallops. However, infection in individual animals can arise without contact, especially where environmental conditions allow existing organisms to invade, or to re-infect (for example, as in herpes infection). Viruses repeatedly crop up in the same place, and there are racing yards which are never free of infection for any length of time. In fact, there are yards where horses in particular boxes are never free of infection, while those in other buildings are frequently healthy.

Move infected horses elsewhere - even, in cases, to different stables in the same yard - and they quickly recover. Until this type of influence is accepted, vaccination is unlikely, ever, to be fully successful, because the diseases are a reflection of stress not just the result of an animal meeting an infectious organism. Even if particular viruses are eliminated, others will step in to fill the void; it is almost inevitable.

Respiratory infection is probably the cause of more trouble to trainers than even lameness. Outbreaks are often related to particular weather patterns. Many yards which suffer at a particular time of year report that their infections disappear when the weather gets warmer. Others only become infected at this time. Research needs to come to terms with this.

Routines

For prevention of respiratory disease in the individual horse, steps should be taken, as:

1)	Make sure each animal is well nourished; malnutrition lowers an animal's resistance to disease.

2)	Ensure stabling is warm, dry and clean.

3)	Treat animals regularly for worms and other parasites, as heavy burdens lower resistance.

4)	Vaccinate for influenza.

For prevention within a yard, where many animals may be kept close together and in relatively close contact, the following steps should be adopted (whilst not neglecting the needs of the individual animal):

1)	Stable hygiene demands proper mucking out and the prevention of ammonia build-up in bedding.

2)	Containers and utensils (for example, feed pots, water buckets and bowls) must at all times be clean. The feed room must be scrupulously clean and the method of distributing food to numbers of horses must be hygienic as well as efficient. If sacks are used, these need to be washed and disinfected regularly.

3)	Hay and straw must be clean, wholesome and free of dust and spores.

4)	Hands, grooming kit and tack must be kept clean. Remember that highly contagious conditions like ringworm can be spread by these means.

5)	Stables between individual horses must be clean and disinfected.

6)	Fittings and surrounds require regular cleaning.

7)	Indoor temperature ranges must be monitored. They are critical to the development or otherwise of infection and are especially important where numbers of horses are kept close together.

8)	There should not be fixed open vents in those buildings housing numbers of horses; adjustable vents can be controlled according to requirements. Never leave any animal in a cross-draught - and do make sure that adjustments at night allow for falling external temperatures.

9)	Increase ventilation if a stable is too stuffy, but without subjecting animals to the effect of chilling. Going from one extreme to the other is not the answer to the problem.

10)	Do not put horses in stables when they are wet - unless it is intended to dry them fully. Do not wash horses excessively or needlessly.

11)	Ensure that the horse is warmly housed. No amount of extra blankets will protect a horse from infection if the basic building temperature is inadequate. Better to have a warmer stable and fewer rugs.

For prevention outside the yard where horses may mingle with others from a variety of locations:

1)   Avoid contact with known infection, especially with animals from yards known to be affected with influenza or strangles.

2)   Avoid using communal tack and ensure the cleanliness and hygiene of stabling used away from home.

3)   Isolate horses returning from events where there has been coughing or other evident sources of infectious disease.

4)   Isolate horses that may have been stressed by long journeys.

For prevention on a day-by-day management system:

1)   Do not move animals in or out of heavily infected areas except under professional advice.

2)   Always isolate sick animals away from others, where possible; especially if they are coughing or have dirty infectious discharges. This helps to dilute infection, reduces the risk to animals in contact, and has a positive effect on recovery. It is important for horse owners to appreciate that the heavier the dose of infectious organism the more likely is it that exposed animals will become infected.

3)   Isolate mares that have aborted; especially keep them well away from horses in training.

4)   In cleaning stables between horses, pay particular attention to dust and cobwebs on walls and ceilings.

5)   Limit human contact between infected animals; also prevent the sharing of containers, implements, etc.

6)   Never allow infection to run its course because this opens the door to build-up and resulting increased virus virulence.

7)   Immediate diagnosis is important; detection is possible in virulent outbreaks through astute observation. Laboratory samples should help confirm the cause.

8)   Immediately reduce exercise levels of affected horses, especially in conditions such as influenza where all exercise of sick animals should be stopped. Ensure adequate ventilation and allow horses to walk out to graze if possible - as long as this does not place other animals at risk. The purpose is to reduce air contamination and foster natural resistance processes. Serious harm can arise from working sick horses.

9)   Disinfect contaminated areas regularly, especially fixtures and fittings.

10)   Any waste food and animal discharges will be a fertile medium for organisms to grow on and need to be cleaned away. If inhaled into the respiratory system these organisms may lead to pneumonia. In the gut they can compete with, and overcome, beneficial organisms; this can lead to acute disturbance in the bowel.

11)   It is wise to have disinfectant containers positioned outside the stables of infected horses, in order that those people entering and leaving can dip their boots. This is good practice in any serious outbreak of disease.

12)   Cold buildings favour the build-up of infection. Evacuate such buildings where possible and turn infected horses out to grass where this can be done without risk to others.

13)   Vehicles going out of, or coming into, a yard may carry infection. During major outbreaks, disinfectant pads should be positioned outside premises - wide enough to take a full revolution of vehicle wheels.

14)   Be constantly vigilant against disease. Be suspicious and treat racecourses, transport, and so on as possible sources of infection. Take added precautions as already advised.

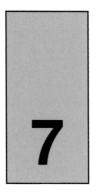

7 Specific Virus Diseases

Equine influenza and herpesvirus infection (rhinopneumonitis) are both considered to be the most important causes of current equine respiratory disease in the United Kingdom and Ireland.

However, it is common that two or more virus species can infect a horse at the same time, or sequentially. This necessarily will affect the clinical picture. It is also considered inevitable that new viruses will be shown to play a role in respiratory disease in time. In these cases, to follow current trends, the effects will be most pronounced in racing animals.

Equine Influenza

In the United Kingdom and Ireland influenza outbreaks have tended to appear in equine populations as a periodic infection of epidemic proportions after relatively disease-free intervals of eight to ten years (although there has been some change in this pattern since the introduction of compulsory vaccination). Vaccinated horses are known to become infected on occasion.

The infection hits old and young alike, and also the highly trained. There is no sign of any natural immunity in the unvaccinated population and acquired immunity (from exposure to infection) in young horses is short lived.

Epidemiology

Many outbreaks of equine influenza occur in two-year-old or three-year-old horses assembled in large groups (for example, in training stables). In virulent outbreaks all groups are affected, even those kept on relatively isolated farms, where horses are small in number yet become infected by passing or neighbouring horses.

Infection is influenced by the level of immunity, the virulence of the virus and the level of exposure - that is, the physical quantity of virus inhaled.

A major outbreak in the United Kingdom and Ireland during 1989 was followed by sporadic cases in the ensuing years. These outbreaks were followed by another serious occurrence, in the summer of 1991. (It has been suggested that foals not affected on studs in 1989 were susceptible when entering training in 1991.) This change of pattern is undoubtedly related to changing viral antigenicity (antibody producing nature) and is disappointing in the face of widespread use of vaccine. It also creates the possibility (in view of further cases in the winter of 1993/94) that the disease is now endemic.

Stress of transport, crowded stabling and poor ventilation are all conducive to infection. The virus survives best in low humidity air and this, as with all airborne viruses, is favoured by low temperatures. Decreased ventilation increases contamination in environmental air samples, further enhancing spread in enclosed housing. Especially dangerous are infected horses showing few clinical signs but shedding virus.

The disease spreads very rapidly, with an incubation period of one to three days, helped by the frequent coughing of affected animals, and subsequent inhalation by other animals.

In droplet form, the virus travels some 20m to 30m at most; however, longer distances of airborne spread have been suspected in some recent situations. The virus is spread by direct human contact, on clothes, implements or by vehicles.

Influenza virus is not long-lived out of the animal and is inactivated by heat, ultraviolet light and disinfectants. Inevitably, there would be little or no infection if horses were not brought into contact with others.

Equine influenza is caused by an orthomyxovirus and is virtually worldwide in distribution; however, in some countries, for example New Zealand and Australia, it has not been recorded to date. In South Africa there was an outbreak in 1986 but it was attributed to the introduction of infected horses into a susceptible population. Influenza is the only equine disease for which there is compulsory vaccination in both the United Kingdom and Ireland at present.

There are three main antigenic strains in present vaccine use. They are known by their manufacturers' references and their names indicate the

geographical source of the original virus isolation. Until recently, these three were the strains used in modern vaccines. They are:
1)   A/equine/1 (Prague '56);
2)   A/equine/2 (Miami '63);
3)   A equine/2 (Kentucky '81).

The first of these strains, A/equine/1 (which has not been recovered since 1979), is also sometimes referred to as H7N7. Similarly, A/equine/2 is also known as H3N8.

Numerous varieties of these antigenic strains are at present circulating, leaving epidemiologists with considerable concerns about updating vaccines (now to be done every four years) and which policies to adopt to limit the incidence of the disease.

A/equine/2 is thought to be more virulent and have a greater affinity for lung tissue than A/equine/1, but to be less antigenic. There is no cross immunity between the two strains; therefore, it is possible (in theory) to have two outbreaks of infection in the same group of horses in a short space of time.

Many other isolates of A/equine/2 - as listed below - are commonly mentioned in the literature:
A/equine/2 (Tokyo '71);
A/equine/1 (Joinville '78);
A/equine/2 (Fontainbleau '79);
A/equine 2 (Newmarket '79);
A/equine/2 (Solvalla '79);
A/equine/2 (Kentucky '81);
A/equine/2 (Johannesburg '86);
A/equine/2 (Tennessee '86)
A/equine/2 (Suffolk '89).

In the United States, A/equine/1 (Prague '56) is the most common H7N7 strain used in vaccines but this subtype also includes A/equine/1 (Newmarket '77). A/equine/2 (Sufolk '89) has recently been included in British vaccines.

Infection in an animal is subject to the following conditions.
1)   Immune status. Not all vaccinated animals are adequately protected in the face of infection and numerous breakdowns have been reported. Better vaccines are now in use and new ISCOM (Immune Stimulating COMplex) vaccines, from which a great deal is expected, are presently available.
2)   Virulence of the virus. This grows as an outbreak gets under way,

creating a situation where even vaccinated animals may not withstand challenge.

3)   The level of exposure. A small dose of virus may be overcome by body defences, but a massive dose will lead to inevitable infection unless there is solid immunity. It is also possible that this situation is affected by virus concentration in inhaled air.

4)   Environmental conditions play a part. Conditions which are too cold or damp will hinder resistance and assist invasion.

5)   Spread is mainly by droplet infection. As an infected horse coughs out virus it is inhaled directly into the respiratory tract of another.

6)   This virus does not live for very long when outside a host but may be carried on contaminated clothing, hands, and so on.

Pathology

When influenza viruses are inhaled, most deposit on the upper airway but some may penetrate more deeply. If there is immunity, these viruses may be neutralised, but this capacity may be lost in the face of heavy challenge, or virulence. The virus invades surface cells in which it multiplies, causing the cells to rupture and spill more virus out into the airways. Spread can occur initially with the help of cilia moving the particles along, spreading throughout the tract in one to three days, but damaging cilia and epithelial cells in the process. Mucociliary clearance is decreased, secretions accumulate in the airways and underlying tissues become inflamed. Large areas of airway epithelium may be denuded, increasing the chance of secondary infection.

It is possible for respiratory cilia to stop working fully as a result of influenza virus.

Symptoms

The clinical picture for horses suffering influenza is the same in many ways as that for humans: temperature variation is sudden in onset and as high as 106 degrees F in some horses.

There is a dry, persistent cough, with rapid spread of infection through a group of horses. The nasal mucous membrane is inflamed as is the lining membrane of the eye (conjunctiva). The horse will be off its food, is depressed in appearance, and develops a dirty nasal discharge. It may be very reluctant to move, and shows great difficulty when asked to do so. The lymph glands in the throat region may be enlarged for a short period. During the acute phase the animal is infectious to others - generally for three to six days, but this may last for as long as eight days. The cough may persist for several weeks, but usually will resolve itself quickly with total rest. Pneumonia is a common secondary complication, especially in foals. Horses may be very flat after infection and it has been found that some are anaemic. When worked or raced during the clinical disease these horses are likely to suffer greatly. Sudden death occurring weeks after an influenza infection has been known; this is considered to be due to an effect on the heart. In such animals there may be ryhthm changes and an increase in the resting heart rate, indicating a need at this time for close clinical supervision. In severe cases, valvular insufficiency and congestive heart failure may occur.

A carrier state has not been detected with equine influenza.

There is improvement in five to seven days in the absence of secondary infection. Resolution of tissue damage takes up to three weeks.

Where vaccinated animals become infected, the symptoms are often less severe and more transient.

Diagnosis

The highly infectious nature of the condition, coughing and nasal discharges are adequate symptoms to support a diagnosis of influenza.

Endoscopic examination reveals pharyngitis, laryngitis and tracheitis for up to a week. The virus can be isolated from infected material at a suitably equipped laboratory. Nasal mucus taken early in the course of the disease is most suitable. Paired serum samples are also used and antibodies are detectable by seven days after infection. These may persist for up to eighteen months.

Blood samples for haematology show a lymphopenia (decrease in the number of lymphocytes) for up to four days, followed by a monocytosis (an increase in the number of monocytes).

An ELISA test is now available for influenza diagnosis, meaning the condition can be confirmed within twenty-four hours; although it does not differentiate between the two subtypes, it is sensitive and rapid.

A clinician would be justified in making a tentative diagnosis on the basis of symptoms, then taking immediate steps within a yard to counter secondary infection, limit movement, introduce hygienic controls and reduce the overall level of infection.

Treatment

Antibiotics are used to control secondary infections. While these will not influence the viral phase of disease, they will help to shorten the overall length of illness and are vital in saving young animals from the effects of bacterial pneumonia. It is advisable to rest affected animals for at least three weeks after recovery from influenza and to restore lost weight fully before returning them to work.

The cycle of events in equine influenza. There is not thought to be a carrier state for the disease although the possibility of mechanical transport (by birds, insects, etc.) is considered

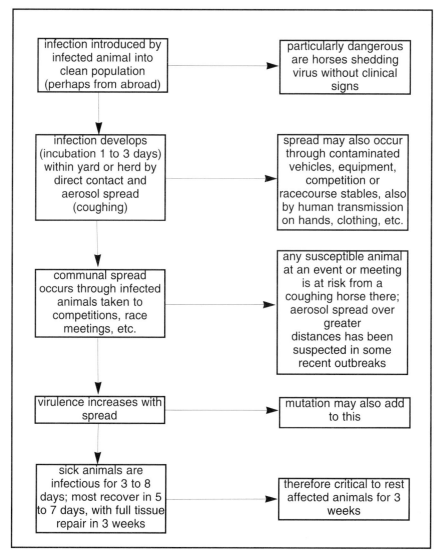

Prevention

In some countries, vaccination is compulsory for all animals taking part in competitions; in others it is voluntary. Vaccination can also be made compulsory by the rules of individual organisations. For example, all horses appearing on racecourses and point-to-point courses in the United Kingdom and Ireland are obliged to have a passport containing details of vaccination that establish current vaccinal status and which must meet standard criteria; the same applies to three-day events, etc.

While there are a number of vaccine types available, no preference is given to any one variety under Jockey Club or Turf Club rules. Neither is any advantage recorded in practice, though oil-based vaccines are more likely to cause local tissue reactions than those which are water-based.

As the vaccine types in use are inactivated virus vaccines they create immunity by setting up a mild clinical reaction (not an infection). Because of this, vaccinated animals should be eased out of work for several days after vaccination.

(New ISCOM vaccines, consisting of inactivated antigens, do not carry this recommendation to rest, though this must be taken in light of the warning of temperature rises after vaccination which occurs in a small number of horses.)

It is also critical that horses suffering the effects of other subclinical viral infections should not be vaccinated until the effects observed have passed off. If vaccination proceeds without observing these precautions, there is a serious risk of complications developing.

It has been suggested that regular updating of vaccine strains may prove effective in controlling influenza in the future. This would mean that the strain or strains causing disease be quickly identified and used to prepare a vaccine. In this way it would be hoped to eliminate the complaints that are made of previous vaccines and the sometimes disappointing protection they offer in the face of infection.

The new generation of ISCOM influenza vaccines, mentioned above, contain inactivated antigens of A/equine/1 (Newmarket) and A/equine/2 (Brentwood). Used in an injection regimen in accordance with Jockey Club regulations, it is suggested that immunity is better and longer lasting than has previously been the case. It is to be hoped that this will prove correct in practice and stand the test of time.

The current regulations for vaccination under Jockey Club rules are as follows:

1)   Two primary injections to be given no less than 21 days, and no longer than 92 days, apart.

2) Horses foaled after 1 January 1980 must have received a first booster injection no less than 150 days, and no more than 215 days, after the second primary injection mentioned in 1) above.

3) Additional booster injections are given at intervals no more than one year apart.

4) None of these injections may have been given within ten days prior to entry onto a racecourse.

Many other bodies (for example, sales companies, stud farms, competition organisations, etc.) adhere to the same, or similar, vaccination requirements.

Control

Equine influenza can spread extremely rapidly; therefore, it is important that all efforts be made to stem the transmission of infection. Essentially, this means a limitation on movement of animals from infected premises and preventing infected animals coming into contact with healthy horses. It also means that infected yards should be closed to the public and individuals in contact with infected horses should not visit places where they might carry infection to uninfected animals, especially on contaminated vehicles or utensils.

As for airborne infections, transmission can be interrupted by eliminating the source and protecting and decreasing the number of susceptible horses by vaccination and isolation. This may well involve administration of booster doses to already fully vaccinated animals, though the procedure has proved disappointing in the past. However, it is to be hoped that better vaccines may eliminate this need in the future.

Stables, transport vehicles and equipment should all be sterilised as appropriate.

Foals are not vaccinated until at least three to six months of age.

Herpesvirus Infection

The disease known as herpesvirus infection, or rhinopneumonitis, has assumed considerable importance in modern equine medicine being identified as a cause of abortion in mares and respiratory infection in horses of all ages.

In some horses herpesvirus infection has also been identified as the cause of staggering, recumbency, and paralysis - indeed, severe outbreaks of paralysis have occurred repeatedly over the past twenty years, mainly on stud farms. The respiratory form of the disease is a major cause of concern to trainers of racehorses.

Epidemiology

Herpes viruses are considered to have a lifetime persistence in the body after infection, though there is some dispute as to the significance of this in horses. While, in particular instances, infection appears to carry on over a lengthy period, horses generally recover fully and are not chronically re-infected for the rest of their lives. However, re-infection may well ensue where resistance is lowered as this group of viruses is adept at exploiting any weakness in body defence systems.

The herpes virus is very fragile in nature and does not persist for very long on exposure. It is spread mainly by droplet infection and direct contact with contaminated material and it is known to spread over wide areas on the wind. In many outbreaks, almost all horses in a yard are infected quickly with the respiratory form of the disease, signs of which can be detected clinically. More insidious development is also known.

We need now to look more closely at the equine herpes viruses and their various disease manifestations.

EHV-1

The generic name for the virus, from which the acronym EHV is derived, is Equid Herpes Virus. EHV-1, the most significant variety, is a major cause both of abortion in mares and upper respiratory disease in horses of all ages. It is a feature of the respiratory form that the infection can be persistent and extend to deeper organs of the body. The liver is commonly affected and the paralytic form of the disease is caused by some strains of this virus entering the central nervous system (it is not yet possible to differentiate a paralytic strain of the virus by laboratory examination). Foals may be weak at birth and die in the first days of life. Pneumonia is a complication in older foals.

The virus is worldwide in distribution and is recognised as having been in existence throughout history.

Pathology and Symptoms

The incubation period is from two to ten days. Transmission may occur by direct contact, and intranasal, oral, conjunctival, intratracheal, vaginal or parenteral inoculation.

The signs in the early stages are very mild and may go unnoticed. Temperature changes may be short-lived (less than twelve hours) or may extend for up to five days and be biphasic (two distinct phases, or showing more than one temperature peak). Virus attachment and penetration into cells is followed by rapid multiplication; vesicles may develop in the trachea and bronchi. Following this the virus enters lymphatics and capillaries and viraemia develops.

Infection is most common in the alveoli of the lungs, but can occur in either the upper or lower tract. The virus can persist in nasal secretions for twenty days post infection. There is evidence of influence of stress in abortions (for example, travel). Fever in infected yearlings may last one week. Horses suffering from herpes infection may cough after exercise, although snorting is a more usual sign.

EHV-1 virus is capable of causing suppression of the immune system of affected animals, and therefore may allow further infection.

Respiratory Form

After incubation, there is frequently a copious watery discharge from the nostrils. Horses will be heard clearing their noses in an explosive way that sprays infected material into the atmosphere rather as it would from an aerosol can. The virus can become very virulent where large numbers of horses are kept together, causing the development of more pronounced symptoms.

High temperatures are possible in the early stages, though their duration may be short-lived - as little as twelve hours - and it is possible to miss them. There is depression, loss of appetite and the glands of the throat may be found to be swollen - though the swelling is not as pronounced as in strangles. The membranes of the nasal passages acquire a typical purple discoloration. The early signs are mild and easily missed.

In foals, pneumonia is a common outcome of this disease. While the general mortality rate is low, deaths are more likely to occur where the organism is virulent and management of a low order.

Systemic and Paralytic Forms

After initial infection there is a tendency for serial cycles of re-infection, though whether these are caused by the same or different viruses is unclear. While re-infection is generally considered most improbable with the same organism (due to the nature of the immune process), it has been suggested that EHV-1 can prove an exception to this. Certainly, on purely clinical grounds, this would appear possible, as the typical condition develops in phases, with repeating disease episodes at about ten-day to two-week intervals. While it is possible that these succeeding phases are caused by secondary viruses, other than EHV-1, it is not proven. A great deal remains to be explained regarding the clinical picture of herpes infection.

Each subsequent episode is marked by a progression of symptoms, with more noticeable temperatures and signs of liver involvement at about seven to ten days from initial infection. The virus grows in the lining cells of blood vessels in the brain and spinal cord, causing haemorrhage and thrombosis. Clinically, it appears there is gradual progression to deeper organs. In some cases, horses are found recumbent without prior warning, but in virtually all of these clinical indications suggest longer-standing disease. Affected horses stagger before going down or may simply be found in the recumbent position. They tend to be bright and may have a good appetite but are simply unable to stand. Others may stand but show impaired nervous function. The condition becomes progressively worse from the point of recumbency; mechanical paralysis occurs due to pressure on nerves, and ulceration of the skin appears if the horse is down for any length of time. The animal may be unable to pass urine and constipation is not unusual.

Muscular complications are a common sequel to the systemic form of the disease and are a suggested consequence of liver damage. Recovering horses may be noted to move badly at work and tend to tie up on fast exercise.

Abortion

Abortion normally occurs in the second half of pregnancy. It is a sequel to respiratory infection and occurs from two weeks to four months thereafter. However, serious outbreaks can lead to abortion storms in which all the normal rules are broken. In such circumstances there may be shortened time intervals - within days of introduction to infection - and thirty-day foetal loss in recently covered mares has been known to occur, though the immediate cause is not yet explained.

Diagnosis

Diagnosis is confirmed by virus isolation or by laboratory examination of

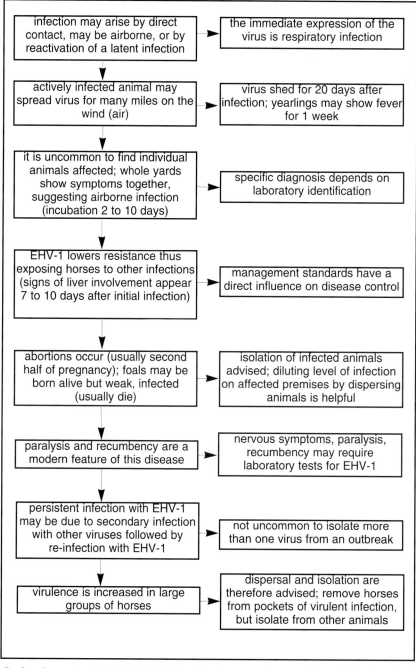

infection may arise by direct contact, may be airborne, or by reactivation of a latent infection	the immediate expression of the virus is respiratory infection
actively infected animal may spread virus for many miles on the wind (air)	virus shed for 20 days after infection; yearlings may show fever for 1 week
it is uncommon to find individual animals affected; whole yards show symptoms together, suggesting airborne infection (incubation 2 to 10 days)	specific diagnosis depends on laboratory identification
EHV-1 lowers resistance thus exposing horses to other infections (signs of liver involvement appear 7 to 10 days after initial infection)	management standards have a direct influence on disease control
abortions occur (usually second half of pregnancy); foals may be born alive but weak, infected (usually die)	isolation of infected animals advised; diluting level of infection on affected premises by dispersing animals is helpful
paralysis and recumbency are a modern feature of this disease	nervous symptoms, paralysis, recumbency may require laboratory tests for EHV-1
persistent infection with EHV-1 may be due to secondary infection with other viruses followed by re-infection with EHV-1	not uncommon to isolate more than one virus from an outbreak
virulence is increased in large groups of horses	dispersal and isolation are therefore advised; remove horses from pockets of virulent infection, but isolate from other animals

Cycle of events with EHV-1. While scientists question persistent infection (and re-infection), symptoms of this disease can exist, especially in racing yards, over very extended periods samples taken from an aborted foetus or dead foal. Also, tracheal washes from horses with the respiratory form of the disease may produce virus growth. Negative results are not necessarily conclusive as EHV-1 can precipitate abortion of a virus-negative foetus on occasion.

In horses which have been previously infected, viral excretion may be minimal and occur for only twenty-four to forty-eight hours, whereas horses affected for the first time will excrete for more than a week. It may be productive, in view of this, to sample younger, previously unexposed horses in a stable.

On endoscopy, the lymphatic tissue of the pharyngeal region shows signs of inflammation and the membranes of both the upper and lower respiratory tract are congested with serous discharges evident.

Blood samples submitted for haematology may show an initial rise in parameters (for example, packed cell volume, haemoglobin, red blood cells) indicating early dehydration. This is very often soon followed by lowering of the same parameters. The white cell count may be marked by an early reduction in numbers, followed by changes in the individual cell averages, with common increases in the monocyte counts.

Paired serum samples are used in diagnosis although the time interval (about two weeks) involved reduces the value of this method.

Treatment

The course of the respiratory disease will not be affected by drugs, though it is vital that infected horses are kept warm and well nourished. Foals may have to be treated with antibiotics to control secondary bacteria, but the warmth of their stables is critical to recovery. Cold and draughts are not easily tolerated. Where there is liver damage, feeding may have to be adjusted to allow for a reduced protein tolerance. Horses must stop work but the value of grass as a tonic should not be underestimated. Spread occurs so rapidly that grazing infected horses is not a serious risk. All horses can graze after the infective stage.

Recumbent horses seldom get back to their feet without help. Slings may be essential - even where these are roughly constructed, they can have the required effect. When horses are down they need turning every few hours to aid their circulation and to limit development of pressure ulcers. Horses in roughly-made slings may easily injure themselves and considerable padding is needed to ensure the chances of this happening are minimised. Fluid levels have to be maintained by administration of electrolyte solutions. Feeding should be laxative in nature to ensure the bowel remains functional.

Aborted mares must be isolated and all contaminated material destroyed. The aborted foetus and afterbirth should be sent to a recognised laboratory for examination.

Prevention

The following measures should be adopted.

1)   Minimise stress caused by overcrowding or poor management.
2)   Prevent introduction of infection from outside and isolate new arrivals if infection is suspected.
3)   Avoid formation of large groups of susceptible animals.
4)   Wean one mare at a time to avoid stress.
5)   Separate pregnant mares from weanlings and transient horses.
6)   Provide well-ventilated clean housing, free of draughts.

The incidence of abortions is thought to be decreased in vaccinated horse populations, but vaccinated animals still become infected if challenged, at a rate of as high as 75 per cent. Abortion storms in vaccinated mares have been attributed to variant virus. Field studies have shown the importance of a well ventilated and clean environment in preventing disease and that tracheal exudate is less in a clean environment than in a poorly-ventilated area with heavy fungus contamination. However, it is important to apply this information intelligently, as a healthy environment is not achieved by creating draughty conditions that favour the propagation of infection.

In most countries, a code of practice exists for this and other diseases. For our purposes in this book we rely on the Code of Practice published in the United Kingdom by the Horserace Betting Levy Board.

It is a complex code aimed at limiting the effects of serious outbreaks. While it is voluntary it is important that it be respected and its recommendations be carefully adhered to.

Regulations are listed for action to be taken when a mare aborts, and steps are advised to limit spread of the disease.

EHV-4

The EHV-4 virus is also known as EHV-1 Subtype 2.

When compared with EHV-1, infection is more prounced in EHV-4 but does not progress beyond the initial respiratory stage. Nor does it generally extend beyond the respiratory system and there is seldom, if ever, abortion in mares.

The main difference between EHV-4 and EHV-1 is the fact that EHV-4 is not associated with large-scale abortion or signs of involvement of the nervous system. Although respiratory membranes become deep purple in colour, there is no jaundice, and no complications involving the muscular system, yet lung involvement is clearer clinically. Temperatures up to 106 degrees F may be noted.

All in all, EHV-4 is less serious than EHV-1, although it is sometimes associated with acute upper respiratory disease in young horses in the first two years of life.

EHV-2

The significance of EHV-2 as a cause of respiratory disease in horses is somewhat controversial. It has been isolated from the respiratory tract of both normal and diseased animals.

EHV-3

The cause of pock (or equine coital exanthema as it is sometimes known) in mares - occurring as blisters on the animal's vulva and surrounding areas - EHV-3 can be venereally transmitted to stallions where it causes the same type of lesion on the penis and sheath. After healing, the damaged areas usually lose their pigment.

Spread also occurs by contact through dirty tail bandages, instruments, utensils, etc.

The condition is mild and the mare usually breeds normally at the next heat period. Stallions may be out of work for a week or more with the infection.

The virus is also known to cause a mild respiratory disease in foals (also causing blisters in the mouth) and yearlings.

The incubation period is from two to six days. The mare's vulva is painful and swollen. Healing of the lesions occurs normally within seven to ten days.

EHV-3 appears to be endemic in the equine breeding populations of the United Kingdom and Ireland and is observed as a regular feature in stud practice.

In outbreaks of herpesvirus infection it is not unusual for more than one species to be isolated at the same time. EHV-1, EHV-4 and EHV-3 have all been known to be present in the same outbreak. This may greatly accentuate the seriousness of the problems produced.

Adenovirus Infection

Except for causing severe, and often fatal, respiratory infections in immune-deficient foals, the role of adenovirus infection in contributing to equine respiratory disease has not been clarified.

Epidemiology

A highly stable and resistant virus, first isolated in 1969, adenovirus is prevalent in horses worldwide.

Most commonly found in Arabian foals with immunodeficiency disease (where it causes fatal pneumonia) adenovirus has also been found in otherwise normal foals with respiratory disease, and in healthy foals. It has also been isolated from mares and racehorses in training. Subclinical infections are not uncommon in unstressed animals.

Adenovirus has been isolated from respiratory infections in the United Kingdom and Ireland, though it is generally only thought to be of real clinical importance in Arabian foals. However, its influence as an opportunist follower to other infections has got to be considered.

Pathology

Adenovirus can infect multiple sites and be excreted in nasal and conjunctival discharges, urine and faeces. Virus is released for a period of up to sixty-eight days after infection.

Symptoms

The incubation period is from three to seven days and recovery is completed within 21 days. Increased respiration rate, fever, nasal and ocular discharges, deep cough, inappetence (poor appetite) and mild depression may occur. Pneumonia and collapse of lung areas are seen at post-mortem examination. Signs reported in mature horses are generally mild and transient.

(A personal observation is that myocarditis - a serious inflammation of heart muscle - does sometimes occur in adult horses in situations where the virus has been isolated. However, it is not possible to say for certain that adenovirus is the cause of this or subsequent heart problems that occur.)

Diagnosis

There is an initial suppression of lymphocytes although these appear in blood samples after a few days. Infection can occur even when foals are immunised by antibodies in colostrum and severe pneumonia can occur even where there are only mild clinical signs (i.e. external signs may not indicate the severity of the condition).

The virus can be isolated early in the disease. Serology is also used.

Treatment and Control

In all neonatal foals the immune status is critical and plasma should be given to deficient animals. This can be done simply by collecting whole blood from the dam (or other suitable donor) into a vessel containing anti-coagulant, allowing the blood to settle, and then drawing off the plasma. The plasma will have separated into a clear column above the cells.

The virus can remain infective for up to 90 days at room temperature so it is important to provide good hygiene to prevent spread between foals as far as this is possible.

Equine Rhinovirus

Equine rhinovirus is also associated with infection of the horse's upper respiratory tract. The incubation period is short, and there is fever for as long as five days. There are no vaccines available.

A picornavirus (a different family, despite the similarity between the titles 'rhinovirus' and 'rhinopneumonitis'), equine rhinovirus is distinct from the herpes virus infections. It is worldwide in distribution and can cause serious infection of young horses, which may cough as a result of infection. Clinical illness may only become apparent when a horse is stressed.

Pathology

There is inflamation of the larnyx and pharynx and secondary infection is common.

Symptoms

There is fever, nasal discharge and a clinical duration of four to five days. There may be ulceration of the nasal mucosa.

Diagnosis

Diagnosis is based on virus isolation and serology. In Europe, antibodies are more commonly found in groups than in single horses. Equine rhinovirus is a less important disease than those others discussed here.

Equine Viral Arteritis

The outbreak of Equine Viral Arteritis (EVA, or pinkeye) in the United Kingdom in 1993 has brought a new significance to this disease, principally because the virus was never previously isolated here. It stresses the importance of disease control between countries and the need for the health status of individual animals to be strictly supervised when movement from infected into clean populations of horses occurs.

Epidemiology

EVA is commonly recognised in North America and Europe. Large horse populations in affected areas formerly experienced epidemics of EVA at intervals of ten to fifteen years.

The disease is caused by a togavirus (family) first isolated in Bucyrus, Ohio in 1953. While the symptoms have been recognised for a century or more, EVA was previously confused with other influenza-like infections.

There are two strains: Bucyrus, which is very virulent, and the milder Penn strain. (The Bibuna strain was isolated in Europe, and in 1964 was found to be identical to the Penn strain.) The condition has been confirmed in Austria, Switzerland, Poland and France, and now the United Kingdom. Occasional suspicious blood titres (antibody development, indicating exposure to the virus) have been taken from animals in other European countries.

The infection which occurred in the United Kingdom was found in six Midlands counties and was quickly and effectively brought under control. While provision was made for the introduction of a new, killed vaccine (initially for use in the affected counties, but now approved for use in all horses throughout the United Kingdom), there is no reason to expect further spread from the initial source - traced to an Anglo-Arab stallion imported from Poland, an eventer that competed throughout the United Kingdom from the time of his arrival in 1992. Mares covered by this stallion became infected through his semen (direct, or venereal, spread) and developed the respiratory form of the disease. These mares spread the infection further (lateral spread).

The distinction between these two types of spread will become clear later in this chapter. A major concern is that EVA causes pregnant mares to abort.

Clinical EVA has not been diagnosed in Ireland.

EVA virus is susceptible to common disinfectants. Its ability to generate disease varies greatly: some infections are inapparent and others severe.

The incidence of clinical disease is high in mares bred to EVA-affected stallions. It is a disease of Standardbred and Saddlebred horses in the United States and only 2 per cent of Thoroughbreds are said to suffer, though there have been serious recorded outbreaks in the Thoroughbred population. Mortality is low and recovery good; however, the disease in previously uninfected populations is likely to be of a severe nature. Deaths have been recorded in young foals.

The transmission of EVA is by direct contact, droplet infection and venereally. The virus can be isolated from saliva, nasal secretions, semen and blood, also urine, faeces and from aborted foetuses. Drinking water, mangers and straw are common sources of infection. The role of biting insects is uncertain.

Epidemics only occur in large, susceptible populations where spread is slower than with influenza.

Freshly infected stallions shed virus from nose and mouth and in their semen for one to three weeks, but 30 per cent or more remain long-term shedders of virus in semen. This chronic carrier state can last for years in stallions.

Freshly infected mares shed virus from nose and mouth for one to three weeks, after which natural immunity develops. Mares and foals may spread the disease in their urine for up to six weeks - but a permanent carrier state in the mare is not thought to occur.

All susceptible mares are thought to become infected when covered by carrier stallions. It is therefore critical that known infected stallions should not cover unprotected mares.

Abortion may occur in mares (most commonly mid to late pregnancy, though possibly at any stage) and abortion rates of 50 to 60 per cent have been reported. Abortion may occur within two weeks of infection (range of 10 to 35 days). An aborted foetus is usually heavily contaminated with virus.

Pathology

After inhalation virus enters the lymphatic system and then the general circulation. The incubation period is seven to nine days venereally, two to fifteen days by respiratory spread. The virus attacks small blood vessels in all parts of the body. This results in impaired circulation, blockage of small vessels and haemorrhage. Oedema also occurs as a result of the activities of the virus.

Symptoms

In the first-ever recorded outbreak there was abortion and influenza-like symptoms. After incubation, there is a serous (watery) nasal discharge (which may become purulent later) and fever may last for up to nine days. Horses may appear sleepy and stagger when moved. They may refuse to eat, can suffer symptoms of depression and their limbs (more commonly hind limbs) and other areas may swell (scrotum, prepuce, udder). There can be diarrhoea, sometimes coughing and respiratory distress - due to inflammation of the digestive and respiratory tracts. Skin rashes and plaques are also a common feature.

Symptoms may be very mild, but fever (up to 106 degrees F) is constant as an early sign and may persist for up to twelve days. There may be excessive discharges from nose and eye and saliva may dribble from the mouth. Mucous membranes may develop a 'brick-red' colour.

Eye symptoms are marked by oedema of the eyelids, conjunctivitis (causing the characteristic pink eye appearance), clouding of the cornea, and sensitivity to light. The conjunctiva is often jaundiced, the pupil constricted, the iris swollen.

Diagnosis

Diagnosis is based on clinical signs, virus isolation and serology. Paired blood samples are taken to detect rising antibody levels. There is also an ELISA test.

Virus can be detected in semen through laboratory examination. Shedding stallions are also detected by their ability to infect susceptible mares.

Vaccination can confuse serology tests.

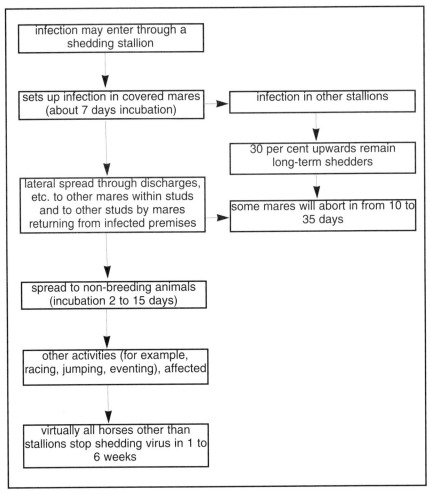

Cycle of events in EVA; it is evident from this that the shedding stallion is a vital influence in the life-cycle of this infection

It should be appreciated that specific diagnosis is essential (especially in populations formerly free of this disease) and must depend on laboratory tests.

Prevention

A modified live virus vaccine has proved effective in the United States, but it is not licensed for use in the United Kingdom and Ireland - where a new killed vaccine was used during the recent outbreak of 1993 and is now available for use subject to official control. At the time of going to press (1994), the controls licensed the new vaccine for full use in the United Kingdom, under supervised control stallions only in Ireland, but all this may change any day.

Isolation is very important in this disease. Movement of horses has to be restricted, and breeding sheds are closed. In the United States, the convention on stud farms is to separate stallions from other stock and mares are walked in for covering when close to ovulation. This reduces the risk of infection, which is further limited by a policy of vaccination. Immunity after infection and vaccination are both considered to be lifelong (not proven with killed vaccine) and vaccinated stallions do not transmit the virus, nor do vaccinated mares develop symptoms after mating with shedding stallions.

It is quite evidently essential in considering prevention of this disease to recognise and control shedding stallions (it is suggested that immediate sexual rest may help prevent the development of a carrier state in stallions freshly infected).

All horses imported from EVA-infected countries should be immediately isolated (for not less than three weeks) and have blood samples taken on arrival and again after ten days. All shedding stallions are positive when blood tested, though all positive stallions are not necessarily shedders. Therefore, a blood-positive stallion is a matter of major concern. Such a stallion would be isolated for not less than thirty days and his semen tested for the presence of virus by both laboratory means and by test mating. Colts out of training intended for use as stallions would be treated in the same way as existing stallions.

Affected or shedding stallions are castrated in some situations. They may also be destroyed or re-exported. Clearly the purpose of any control measure is to prevent the introduction of infection. However, as has happened in 1993, it is vital that any infection that evades normal controls should be quickly and effectively contained. Therefore, isolation of known infected and all contact animals is a priority.

Aborted foetuses (and their membranes), being a potent source of virus, capable of infecting other mares that may sniff them or of contaminating grazing ground where this might happen, should be submitted for laboratory examination; complete disinfection of the contaminated area must be carried out in its wake.

Vaccination is an evident adjunct to this.

There is a Common Code of Practice covering this disease which should be adhered to. As current European Community conditions allow free movement of horses within the countries of the community, there is an onus on the individual importing a horse from known infected countries to protect the common interest by taking full precautions. This is particularly important, especially when it is considered that the animal responsible for the recent outbreak (1993) in the United Kingdom came with a certificate of freedom from this disease which later proved to be incorrect. Similar precautions must also be taken when importing semen.

The Common Code of Practice is published by the Horserace Betting Levy Board and is available from the breeders' associations in France, Germany, Ireland, Italy and the UK.

In Ireland, EVA is a notifiable disease; this means that any outbreak would involve restrictions on movement of horses and could cause the cancellation of equestrian events, including race meetings. Finally, to prevent export complications with animals vaccinated against EVA, it is advisable to blood test prior to vaccination in order to verify a disease-free status.

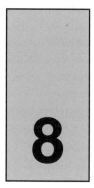

8 Bacterial, Fungal and Parasitic Lung Disease

From a clinical viewpoint, the essential difference observed between viral and bacterial disease is in the severity and nature of symptoms. Bacteria are frequently involved in localised infection of damaged or debilitated tissues, in any location, although they are also capable of causing general infection by entering the bloodstream (septicaemia).

In the respiratory tract, bacterial infections are marked by invasion of tissues of the pharyngeal region (pharyngitis), as occurs in strangles, or by outright pneumonia, which may cover extensive areas of lung tissue and can include the pleura (pleurisy).

Pleuropneumonia involves infection of both pleura and lung tissue; bronchitis is inflammation of the bronchi; bronchiolitis inflammation of the bronchioles; and tracheitis inflammation of the trachea. Rhinitis (inflammation of the nasal passages) suggests that rhinopneumonitis involves both the upper and lower respiratory tract.

Bacterial Diseases

Although there are exceptions, temperatures are generally higher and more persistent in bacterial infections. Pneumonia (as observed clinically) is less common in the adult horse than in other species of animal, but death is more likely to result from established bacterial pneumonia than from most equine viruses presently encountered. Bacterial pneumonia may arise secondary to any form of tissue destruction, such as that caused by toxic smoke or inhaled chemical poisons, for example. It may also follow asymptomatic viral or mycoplasmal (a variety of bacteria) infections.

Bacterial pneumonia can also arise when body resistance is lowered through stress or debility.

Infections may involve a mixture of bacteria or can be caused by one predominant type. Treatment in many such cases is with broad spectrum antibiotics and with every effort made to resolve the underlying tissue weakness. If the respiratory epithelium is mechanically damaged - for example, by toxic fume inhalation - it might be necessary to continue antibacterial treatment until it has had time to recover.

Bacterial infections commonly occur in foals and particularly in the neonatal period. This is due, very often, to poor immune status, usually caused by a failure of passive transfer from the dam in colostrum.

There are, of course, a number of bacterial diseases (an example is tuberculosis which is rare in horses; where it does occur it is sometimes caused by the avian strain of the organism). Restrictions on space in this book does not allow description of them all. However, we discuss below the most significant bacterial conditions usually encountered.

Strangles

Strangles is caused by *Streptococcus equi* and is restricted to equines. It is highly contagious and the principle symptoms of the condition are a thick

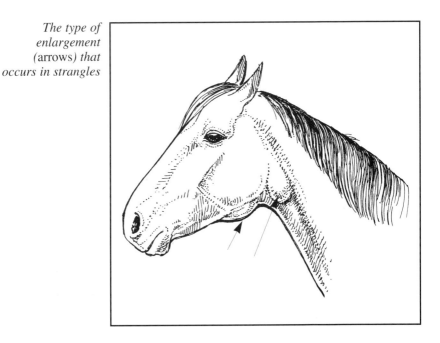

The type of enlargement (arrows) *that occurs in strangles*

purulent discharge from the nostrils and gross enlargement of the glands under the back of the jaw. It can infect horses of all ages, after which immunity (of uncertain duration) develops.

Epidemiology

A virulent organism, *S. equi* is not easy to control once symptoms have begun to show. The organism enters tissues in the pharyngeal area and is spread through infected discharges. This may occur from animal to animal, but also through human transport on hands and equipment. Infected glands may break out and discharge the organism for weeks on end.

The disease may survive on wooden surfaces for seven to nine weeks depending on temperature; elimination of prolonged outbreaks requires resting contaminated areas for at least this long together with thorough disinfection.

A carrier state exists. In most horses nasal shedding ceases after six weeks, but individual animals can shed for up to eight months. Infection is often introduced by a horse that is either incubating the disease or is asymptomatic.

Morbidity can be as high as 100 per cent, but is usually lower. Mortality is low.

Pathology

The organism produces abscesses in the lymphoid follicles of the horse's pharynx. The abscesses mature quickly and drain; infection spreads to the lymph nodes which then become swollen from abscess formation and break out, usually externally through the skin.

Symptoms

Strangles can affect horses of any age. Clinical signs appear from two to twenty days after exposure, though the usual incubation period is in the region of seven to ten days (shorter in established outbreaks). The first signs are an evident soreness of the throat with difficulty in swallowing. Horses make characteristic throaty sounds and may be unable to swallow or drink. The temperature rises to as high as 106 degrees F and within days a watery discharge turns purulent at the nostrils. The submaxillary, and other, lymphatic glands begin to swell. These swellings become hot, tense and painful, and may be present on one or both sides of the jaw. Other glands in the region may also become affected. The glands tend to burst and discharge pus and this may be a prolonged process, though complete recovery after gland discharge is usual.

There is often depression and some horses may cough, although a barking sound that indicates pain in the pharyngeal area may not amount to a true cough. The glands may burst inwardly as well as externally and can cause pneumonia if purulent material is inhaled into the lungs. The gutteral pouch may also become affected, as may other structures in the area.

In an atypical form of the disease symptoms are less severe, although there can be a purulent nasal discharge, even without enlarged glands. Symptoms last from as little as one week to over two months.

Bastard strangles occurs when there is spread of infection from regional to other lymph nodes (for example, of lungs, liver, spleen, kidney, brain and skin). Joints and tendon sheaths may also become affected. This form of the disease is usually difficult to cure and may lead to death.

Purpura haemorrhagica can occur as a sequel to strangles. It is marked by fever, oedematous swelling of the limbs, head, and lower body surfaces. Small haemorrhages appear on mucous membranes and weals may occur all over the body. There may be kidney problems and colic. This condition is an immune complex disease and can occur after infections other than strangles.

The disease can be very debilitating and horses may take a long time to recover condition fully after an attack. Foals that are infected are more likely to die from septicaemia, especially in the first weeks of life.

Diagnosis

Signs of painful throat with difficulty in swallowing are typical of early strangles infection and should be taken as a warning if seen in more than one animal at a time. The full course of the disease, with discharging glands and so on, is easily recognised. Occasional cases of similar type infection occur in individual animals - not in whole herds.

The *S. equi* organism can be isolated from infected material at a laboratory and positively identified. Nasal swabs may be a better source of the organism than pharyngeal; and the organism can be grown from swabs taken directly from lymph nodes.

Treatment

Infected horses should be kept warm and out of draughts. Soft food and mashes are given to those that have difficulty swallowing.

While penicillin is effective against the causal organism its use in an outbreak is of questionable value and, it has been suggested, may lead to development of 'bastard strangles'. However, a decision on the use of antibiotics will be made considering all factors involved and what is best in the particular situation. Although vaccines have been produced, they can cause tissue reactions and the immunity they create is limited; for these reasons, they are not widely used.

Any animal with signs of internal spread, or pneumonia, will require rigorous antibiotic and other supportive treatment. Generally, in these cases, the prognosis is not good.

Control

Owing to the highly contagious nature of strangles, great care must be taken to isolate infected animals and prevent spread within a yard. If the first affected animal has managed to infect a pasture, it is then advisable to suspend use of that pasture and isolate all other animals which have been grazing it. Fresh infection in stabled horses can occur through direct contact, and by human assistance; horses introduced into already contaminated premises may pick up infection from most surfaces. Tight control on each of these sources is therefore essential. Discharges from infected animals are potentially dangerous, so hands, clothing and footwear are in need of scrupulous attention. There should be containers of strong disinfectant outside stable doors to be used by all who enter and leave. Where possible a person attending an infected horse should not attend any other, or the animal should be seen to last of all. There should be individual food and water buckets for each animal; it is imperative that stables be rigorously scrubbed and disinfected between horses.

Infected horses should be isolated for at least six to eight weeks after all symptoms have disappeared.

Foals born to immune mares are resistant for up to three months.

After infection, animals which are a possible source of danger to others may be swabbed on a regular basis to check for excretion of the causative organism. A sequence of negative swabs over a three to six week period might be considered prudent.

Streptococcus zooepidemicus

One of the most common equine bacterial isolates, *Streptococcus zooepidemicus* has at least fifteen different serology types (serotypes). The relevance of the different types to clinical disease and immunity is not yet fully known. It is isolated from the upper respiratory tract and tracheal washes of healthy horses and has also been isolated post-mortem from the trachea.

Pathology

S. zooepidemicus cannot invade intact mucous membranes and therefore pre-existing damage is necessary for infection. It is probably most important as a secondary invader when host susceptibility is increased by viral infection and possibly by stress such as transport or intensive exercise. Severe respiratory diseases such as pleuropneumonia are known to occur more frequently following transport when compared with other forms of stress.

When a susceptible horse inhales *S. zooepidemicus* organisms, infections of the upper respiratory tract such as sinusitis and lymph node abscesses may occur. The lower respiratory tract can become infected, leading to diffuse or focal pneumonia, abscesses or pleurisy.

Clinical signs depend on the horse's immune status, the amount of infection and whether the upper or lower respiratory tract is more adversely affected. Neonatal infections may occur through the navel and cause septicaemia.

Symptoms and Diagnosis

Depression, fever, anorexia and mucopurulent nasal discharge are common clinical signs of infection. The submaxillary glands may be enlarged, sinusitis may occur, or pneumonia and pleurisy develop. Abnormal sounds may be heard on auscultation.

Isolation of the organism is the basis of diagnosis and this is easily grown from submitted material at a laboratory.

Treatment

Treatment is based on sensitivity tests and the use of the appropriate antibiotics. Drainage and flushing of infected areas, such as the sinuses or gutteral pouch, may be necessary.

Streptococcus pneumoniae

A significant cause of pneumonia in neonatal and elderly humans, the

Streptococcus pneumoniae organism is frequently isolated from respiratory tract samples in horses. It is the possible cause of pneumonia, pleurisy and pericarditis.

Rhodococcus equi

Formerly called *Corynebacterium equi*, the *Rhodococcus equi* organism causes pneumonia in foals, though rarely in older horses, on a worldwide basis. It was first isolated in 1923. An incidence of infection as high as 17 per cent worldwide has been reported with a mortality rate of 80 per cent. Mortality is highest in foals of about two months old, but the condition can occur in animals of up to six months or more. Management and environmental factors play major roles in determining the magnitude of the challenge, and therefore affect the prevalance of the disease.

The ability of foals to withstand this infection is dependent on both the degree of environmental contamination and the effectiveness of immune transfer from the dam. *R. equi* is considered to be maintained as part of a normal gut flora, and foals may become infected by eating droppings (coprophagia). It is also present in soil, even in land not grazed by horses, and most likely to be encountered in the warmer months of the year.

The prevalence of infection increases with dusty environments and dry weather, and the organism is not affected by direct sunlight. Foals kept in stables are considered to be more at risk of inhaling the organism than when at pasture.

Pathology

The main routes of infection are the digestive and respiratory tracts. Ingestion is the chief route of exposure in all foals, but rarely leads to respiratory disease. Inhalation causes disease in the foal's respiratory tract, especially the lungs.

When ingested, the organism penetrates the bowel and causes abscess formation in local lymph nodes. In the lungs, abscesses are formed in lymph nodes and in lung tissue.

Although infection is thought to occur in the neonatal period, signs are often not noticed until the foal is more than one month old.

Symptoms

Two clinical forms of *R. equi* infection exist: subacute and chronic.

In the subacute form foals die within days of showing respiratory distress. The lesions in these are chronic in nature although the disease is said to be subacute (i.e. the development of abcesses in glands occurs over a period of time but a clinical crisis then occurs resulting in death, creating the impression of a subacute nature to the disease).

In the chronic form, pneumonia and unthriftiness progress for weeks or months, and foals that survive may have permanently damaged lungs. Some foals are found dead, with lung abscesses located on post-mortem. Others have high fever, rapid deep breathing, and discoloured membranes. They are usually off suck and weak, may be anxious and may not lie down. Nasal discharge and coughing are inconsistent. Severely affected foals die within days despite treatment. Others with the disease may show a more chronic course, of prolonged or recurrent fever, depression, heavy breathing, loss of condition and will eventually become unthrifty. Coughing, if present, is usually soft and deep. Some sufferers will have enlarged joints, with or without evident lameness.

Diagnosis

Haematology may reveal an increased white blood cell count, but this is not specific for *R. equi* infection. Radiography is used to identify lesions in the lungs. The organism can be isolated from material taken directly from lesions or from tracheal exudates. False negatives can occur due to the organism not growing on culture. This occurs because the bacterium may be contained within defensive blood cells and are, therefore, cocooned as within a shell, and not able to grow on the culture medium (nutrient) provided. Results of ELISA tests have been variable. Other blood and antibody tests can be equally unsatisfactory.

Treatment and Control

The organism responds to certain antibiotics, although infections of this nature are naturally resistant and, even in successful cases, treatment may be very prolonged. Plasma from the mare is used to good effect in early treatment and affected foals require nursing, adequate warmth and nourishment. If breathing is too laboured the foal will die, or be put down. Prolonged intravenous feeding is not a practical proposition in most cases.

Prevention

Foals should be housed in well ventilated, but warm, dust-free areas. Dirt paddocks are best avoided, as is crowding, especially around congested stable areas. Manure should be removed from paddocks, and all foals kept off endemic farms. Infected pastures should be avoided. Sandy or dusty areas of grazed pastures should be fenced off.

Sick foals are usually isolated. All in-contact foals are examined two or three times a week, including taking temperatures and examining the lungs. It is important to carry out post-mortem examinations on all dead foals.

Bordetella bronchiseptica

This bacterium attaches to airway surfaces where it may cause acute inflammation, with mucus secretion and inhibition of mucociliary clearance.

Fungal Infections

Fungi such as *Aspergillus* thrive in dusty hay and straw and are important as the cause of localised infections in areas such as the gutteral pouch. Fungal spores can also be the cause of allergic tissue reactions in COPD and similar conditions.

Bedding down horses on straw increases the concentration of respirable dust many times, depending, naturally, on the quality of the straw. Horses in old barns are more exposed to fungi than those in new clean buildings.

However, there has to be a practical aspect to this kind of information. Where there has been a prolonged build-up of spores in a building, removal, or a significant reduction, can be achieved by thorough cleaning.

Parasitic Respiratory Infections

In addition to bacterial and fungal infections, parasitic respiratory infections also occur. Again, space restrictions in this book means we cannot examine them all here. A selection follow.

Lungworm

A parasitic respiratory infection, the lungworm, *Dictyocaulus Arnfield,* can be the cause of chronic coughing in horses, especially where it has had access to land grazed by donkeys. Adult lungworms live in the bronchi of the horse, where eggs are laid on the mucous covering. From here they are carried by mucociliary clearance to the pharynx, and then passed out in the faeces.

Donkeys and mules act as reservoir hosts, seldom showing symptoms although they infect pastures with eggs. The eggs hatch within forty-eight hours of reaching the ground into a first stage larva. After a further forty-eight hours this larva moults and becomes the second stage larva, which matures to an infective stage in about six to seven days. Once these are eaten they migrate through the tissues to the lungs where they mature into adults and lay eggs after thirteen weeks.

The horse and pony are not natural hosts for this worm and are often incapable of infecting others. This occurs because the worm may fail to develop to the egg-laying stage in the bronchi of particular animals.

First stage larvae can live for seven weeks in warm soil, but cannot over-winter or withstand excessive heat or cold. They thrive on warm humid conditions.

Diagnosis

While the presence of a chronic dry cough may create suspicion of lungworm infestation, positive diagnosis is made when eggs are identified in faecal samples. However, a negative result is not conclusive and it may be difficult to establish an opinion on this basis; if lungworm is suspected, it is best to dose with an effective drug and observe the response.

Treatment

Ivermectin is effective against lungworm. Fenbendazole is also successful when used at twice the recommended dose rate.

Roundworm

Another parasitic respiratory infection, roundworm (*Parascaris equorum*) is common in the horse and donkey.

This roundworm is a yellowish white colour and can be up to 35cm in length when fully grown; it is pointed at one end and about as thick as a knitting-needle.

Roundworms are the cause of considerable trouble in foals, where they may accumulate and virtually block the small bowel. In adults, they do not have the same significance.

The female worm lays her eggs in the animal's gut. The eggs are passed out in the horse's droppings and once on the pasture a larva grows within each egg - which is very weather resistant - and these are eaten by the next host. In the gut the eggs then hatch and the larvae penetrate the intestinal wall and migrate throughout the horse's internal organs to the lungs. They find their way into the trachea, from which they are coughed up and then swallowed. Returning to the gut, they grow into mature worms.

Because of this life-cycle, *Parascaris* infestations may cause clinical respiratory disease in the foal.

Symptoms and Diagnosis

Unless present in large numbers there is little external disturbance, the diagnosis being made when the eggs are seen in samples of the horse's droppings. Young animals with heavy infestations will be poor in condition, with staring coats and pot bellies.

Foals of eight to ten months sometimes cough, lose weight and tend to develop serous or mucoid nasal discharges. Symptoms may occur in the pre-patent period before eggs are laid.

Treatment

Roundworms are susceptible to most modern worm drugs. The control of pasture contamination is important, meaning regular removal of faeces.

Redworm

Redworms, strongyles - especially the large strongyles - migrate through body tissues as a part of their natural life-cycle. In this way, they may also be responsible for provoking lung disease.

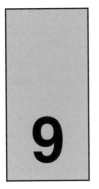

9 Non-infectious Lung Disease

As the title implies, 'non-infectious' diseases of the respiratory tract are diseases in which there is no direct infection of tissues by bacteria or viruses. However, as in COPD, other types of reaction to organisms may be involved.

Chronic Obstructive Pulmonary Disease

The acronym COPD is widely used today when referring to chronic obstructive pulmonary disease; however, it is still known by numerous other names (for example, heaves, broken wind, chronic emphysema, chronic bronchitis, chronic bronchiolitis, recurrent airway obstruction and hay sickness).

COPD is commonly associated with fungal spores and hyphae, pollens and dust in hay and straw and is a complex syndrome with symptoms ranging from exercise intolerance to laboured exhalation, nasal discharge, cough and weight loss. It is, too, one of the most frequently diagnosed non-infectious conditions of the equine respiratory system, increasing in incidence as horses get older, though commonly seen in younger animals, especially those in training.

The disease is mainly associated with the indoor horse, as symptoms are generally reduced or absent when affected animals are at grass. The fungal spores and pollens that often precipitate the condition can saturate dust in stables and be presented to susceptible animals when bedding or hay is shaken up and even when dust on walls and ceiling are agitated by coughing.

COPD can lead to emphysema (a pathological accumulation of air in lung tissues) which is marked by wheezing, increased breathing rate, and by difficulty in taking breath. The wall of the horse's abdomen lifts with each inhalation of air and there is a marked line (the heave-line) at the bottom of the ribs and abdomen. A double movement marks exhalation, due to contraction of the abdominal muscles as the animal attempts to empty the lungs of air.

There are all grades of COPD, varying from the mild to the suffocating. Many affected horses still manage to perform perfectly useful duties despite it. Also, with the advent of some modern drugs, the influence of the condition has been brought under greater control.

Causes

Although allergy is thought to be a prime cause, there may be numerous other factors involved. However, symptoms can easily be produced by exposing horses to musty hay or straw, although some recover fully from this, even without treatment, while others do not. It is known also to be triggered by other factors found in hay besides spores and pollens.

Viruses may cause long-term lung damage and cause the same type of

In COPD the horse's nostrils are flared, chest expanded; there is usually a heave line (arrowed). *The animal may have a chronic cough*

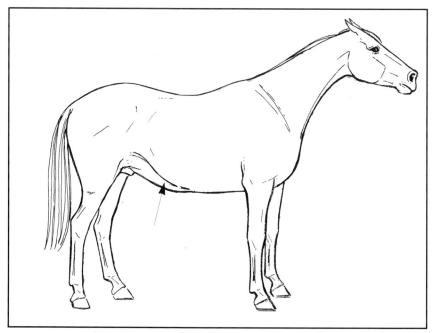

syndrome. Their influence may lead to airway narrowing, thereby reducing ventilation and leaving the animal more susceptible to COPD.

There is a genetic influence recognised in human asthma. Although this is suspected in COPD it has not been proven in the horse.

Pathology

In affected lung regions, the airways are plugged with mucus. The lining membranes are thickened and inflamed, and thus the effective available ventilation space becomes reduced.

Lung compliance and elasticity are gradually lost during the course of this condition, so that there is an increased resistance to air evacuation. This is accentuated by spasm of muscle in the bronchi.

Affected horses are more sensitive to irritants like smoke, ammonia and dust. The cough reflex is triggered by stimulation of three different types of receptor. These respond to mechanical stimulation, foreign materials (such as dust and fungal spores) and chemical substances (like ammonia and toxic gases). Airway inflammation, as exists in COPD, exposes these receptors and this in turn leads to chronic coughing from otherwise innocuous stimuli.

Heart problems may ensue from chronic respiratory disease of this nature.

Symptoms

Affected horses first suffer from a lowered exercise tolerance. In a racehorse, this will show up as reduced performance at work or racing. Coughing may not be noticed, although the resting respiratory rate is increased, recovery after work is extended, and a watery nasal discharge may be seen.

As the condition advances, breathing becomes more laboured and the performance of the animal suffers accordingly. The membranes of the nose and eye become notably congested and coughing - a deep abdominal cough - may become persistent. Loud wheezing sounds are heard from the lungs and efforts to exhale are marked.

Symptoms may develop very slowly and the first sign noticed can be a fall-off in performance. However, even at this stage, the character of breathing at rest will certainly have changed and first indications of an abdominal element to expiration will be detectable. Early signs of a heave-line will be seen if carefully looked for.

The condition may progress gradually to a point where a horse at rest is in evident oxygen debt, in which case it may no longer be practical to keep the horse stabled.

Diagnosis

COPD is distinguished from other respiratory conditions which increase breathing rate. There is no temperature, no infectious discharge, and the animal is often bright and in good condition despite its very poor exercise tolerance.

It is often necessary to exercise the horse first in order to increase the volume of lung sounds, for auscultation in early cases. Wheezes and crackles are common. There is an enlarged lung field in advanced cases (noticeable at rest) because the horse needs more ventilation space.

Endoscopy of the upper airway is usually normal, though exudate arising from the trachea may coat the pharynx. In COPD, introduction of the endoscope into the trachea may provoke coughing, suggesting an irritable airway. Yellow viscous material may be present. With longer endoscopes, the airways do not appear to be inflamed, though exudate is present.

Radiography has not proved to be helpful in diagnosis. Washings taken from the lower airways contain neutrophils. ELISA tests are available to detect the allergic status of horses.

Treatment

Clenbuterol is useful in controlling the symptoms of COPD in milder cases. Its effect is to relieve spasm of lung tissues and to aid the removal of exudates. Many other useful drugs are also available (for example, sodium cromoglycate which is given by inhalation, mainly as a preventive). Corticosteroids have been used to reverse the symptoms, but are not a long-term solution to the problem. Their potential side-effects often preclude their use. Ideally, effective drugs relieve airway spasm, clear accumulated discharges and reduce inflammation of lung tissues.

Control

Management of COPD horses is a matter of prime importance and will follow the pattern listed below.
1)   The animal should be kept in an atmosphere free of dust.
2)   Attention must be paid to the quality of hay fed. It should be well made, dust-free and possibly damped. Some horses suffering from COPD are unable to tolerate hay and may be fed exclusively on grass or haylage.

3)   Straw bedding should be replaced completely by shavings or paper.

4)   If other horses in the immediate vicinity are not kept in the same manner they will serve to promote the condition by stirring allergens into the atmosphere.

5)   A great deal has been written about ventilation for horses with COPD. While it has to be appreciated that any animal having difficulty getting oxygen needs plenty of air, draughty conditions will inhibit the natural defences of the respiratory system and encourage infection. It is not difficult to marry the two needs together in order that a horse can be adequately ventilated and still warm. While this is often questioned by academics, it is a reality of clinical disease control. Tradition has tended to move away from what is acceptable to the horse, and the consequence is increased disease incidence.

6)   COPD can often be life-lasting and affected animals need to be protected from its effects continually. However, modern therapies coupled with good management allow many horses to live full, competitive lives despite it.

7)   Badly-affected horses may be trained from field shelters and kept on a diet primarily of grass and dust-free rations.

8)   Rest may be indicated on occasion to allow the resolution of inflamed tissues.

9)   The onset of COPD is sometimes associated with feeding new batches of hay. This should be avoidable, although some individual horse owners are unable to gauge hay quality.

10)   Horses with severe respiratory allergies require identification of the source in order that COPD can be treated. Though tests tend to be flawed, nonetheless they are now commercially available and used to identify causative allergens. These tests are expensive and results are not always satisfactory.

Exercise Induced Pulmonary Haemorrhage

The acronym EIPH is used today to describe exercise induced pulmonary haemorrhage, a condition that has been known to exist in horses through-out history. EIPH is marked by bleeding from the lungs and it occurs most commonly during racing. While signs of blood are often detected at the nostrils, this is not inevitable.

Recent opinion suggests that a large percentage of racehorses suffer some degree of bleeding during races, even where there is no apparent external sign. The incidence is put as high as 75 per cent in Thoroughbreds, though is less in other breeds. It is suggested that most horses in training experience the condition at some time or other. There is no sex difference but there is an increasing incidence with age.

The influence of the condition on performance is variable, and some trainers believe it appears sporadically. However, some animals do bleed persistently and are in evident pain after it has happened. Although some may show signs of bleeding after races in which they have performed well, bleeding more often interferes with the performance itself.

Pathogenesis

While the exact cause of EIPH is unknown, bleeding usually occurs from areas of the lung previously affected by infection or allergic conditions. It is suggested that bleeding occurs in normal healthy horses but the recognised increase in incidence after virus disease puts this in question. The most common area affected is the upper part of the caudal (hindmost) lobe of each lung. It can be suggested that the immediate cause is the demand for added oxygen, usually in the latter part of a race, and results from dynamic forces being applied to lung tissues which are unable to respond due to earlier disease.

In such lungs there is a loss of elasticity and compliance, thereby reducing ventilation. It is also possible that the source of the blood is from currently inflamed lung areas.

Symptoms and Diagnosis

A horse that is not showing external signs of bleeding, but is suspected of suffering from EIPH nonetheless, should be examined by endoscope after

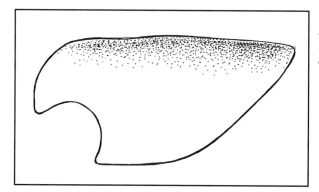

The dappled area shows the part of the lung most commonly affected in EIPH

exercise. Fresh blood may be located in the trachea and bronchi. This examination may be carried out where the horse has stopped suddenly in a race but exhibited no external signs of bleeding. A negative result does not necessarily mean the horse has not bled. In positive cases, blood will normally be seen for up to 90 minutes after exercise - but it may even be detectable for several hours. Microscopic evidence of bleeding can be found in tracheal washes for up to 150 days after a bleeding episode.

More recently, radiography and thermal imaging have been used to identify the areas from which blood has originated.

In the United States, some racing authorities require a signed affidavit from a licensed veterinarian stating that the horse has suffered from EIPH, before allowing pre-race medication to be administered.

In some horses, swallowing after exercise is caused by blood returning from the lungs. Coughing is not a specific sign, but difficult or laboured breathing may occur. In severe cases, the horse will display a low level of pain and areas of the lung may be found to be abnormal on ausculation. The animal may be disinclined to move and not wish to reach to the floor for its food or water.

Treatment

It is important to eliminate other possible causes, especially if no blood is located. Where bleeding occurs as a result of allergy or infection, these conditions will have to be treated individually. Where possible, a spell at grass is useful, especially for horses which repeatedly break blood vessels. In some countries, the lungs of affected horses are flushed out using anti-inflammatory and anti-fungal drugs, following which the animal is turned out. It is hard to be objective about results.

While many proprietary drugs are in current use, their influence, with very few exceptions, is limited. In the United States, frusemide is allowed for use in racehorses by some authorities. However, it is not permitted in European racing. This drug is a diuretic and there is no accepted reasoning for why it should work, though there is a suggestion that frusemide has an effect on blood volume and hence blood pressure. Other suggestions consider an influence on intestinal fluid volume to be a factor.

Controversy also surrounds the question of whether frusemide is performance enhancing or not. While there is no rational reason why it should be, there is little doubt that some horses do improve dramatically while under its influence. However, many other natural therapies can have dramatic effects on horses which may appear clinically normal (for example, the response to fluid therapy of horses which are dehydrated).

While frusemide is known to reduce the incidence of bleeding episodes, it has no effect on the long-term development of the disease and its influence is limited to a single race.

There are many other forms of treatment in use, although few show any significant influence on EIPH.

Prevention

Horses that bleed persistently usually improve after a break from training, and ideally are given an extended period at grass. It would certainly appear that the incidence of EIPH is reduced after extended grass rest, and some horses do not bleed again.

If a horse is a 'whistler and roarer', suffering from ILH, it is possible that the reduction of air-intake has a positive effect on EIPH. Surgery may alleviate the symptoms.

Any condition that reduces ventilation space in the lungs is likely to increase the prospect of EIPH. For this reason, bronchodilators are sometimes used as a preventive.

Nasal Bleeding

Spontaneous nasal bleeding, or epistaxis, in horses not at exercise or at rest will vary in quantity from light to profuse. Sometimes infection of the gutteral pouch is the cause and bleeding can be serious and may even cause death.

Bleeding can also occur from other sites in the respiratory tract, and may be as a result of infection or growths.

Treatment

Local treatment of epistaxis is not easily achieved. However, many instances are isolated and do not threaten future wellbeing. Bleeding from the gutteral pouch may be continuous, profuse and life-threatening. Surgical interference may be the only approach, but this may prove disappointing.

10 | Conditions of the Pharynx and Larynx

Mechanical conditions of the upper respiratory tract are most commonly represented by laryngeal hemiplegia, the common name for which is whistling and roaring - or, as mentioned earlier, ILH. Other conditions, of course, are equally important, such as dorsal displacement of the soft palate (DDSP).

Those conditions listed earlier in this book (i.e. all those mentioned in Chapter 4) are now mentioned in general sales catalogues, especially in the United States, and relate to horses which may be rejected after sale. It is, therefore, important that people who are involved with horses, in whatever capacity should have some understanding of these various conditions and what they mean in relation to airway obstruction and soundness.

ILH

The condition known as ILH (or, to give it its full name, idiopathic laryngeal hemiplegia) is thought to affect as many as 5 per cent of all yearlings at sales. It is caused by changes in the structures of the horse's larynx.

While the exact cause of ILH is not known, the symptoms are related to identifiable changes in the recurrent laryngeal nerve - usually of the left side only.

The larynx is a hollow, rigid structure with walls made up of cartilages united through joints and ligaments, lined on the inside by a continuation of the mucous membrane of the throat and windpipe. This membrane is raised to form a pair of vocal cords each of which enfolds the underlying vocal ligament. During inhalation the vocal cords are removed from the centre line of the larynx, to allow free access of air to the lungs. Both relax on expiration and are critical organs of voice.

The movements of the larynx are controlled by a number of small muscles. They receive their nerve supply through the recurrent laryngeal, a slender nerve that ascends either side of the neck. Each of these nerves follows a tortuous path. At the base of the neck, on the right side, the nerve winds round a small artery and then runs back up the jugular groove along with the common carotid artery to the larynx. The left nerve passes back even further into the chest before it winds round the large main artery at the base of the heart and then follows the same course as the right nerve up the neck.

As whistling and roaring are due to partial paralysis of the left vocal cord, and this is related to damage in the left nerve, various theories abound as to how this damage occurs.

The most popular belief is that the damage is physical, due to stretching of the nerve as it passes round the artery at the base of the heart. This has never been fully proven.

There is a recognised genetic link and it is strongly advised that horses suffering from the problem should not be bred from.

While there is also a suggestion that ILH may follow infection, this has

The normal larynx of the horse (left); *and* (right) *atrophy of the left side* (arrowed) *of the larynx . This left-sided paralysis is common in horses suffering from ILH*

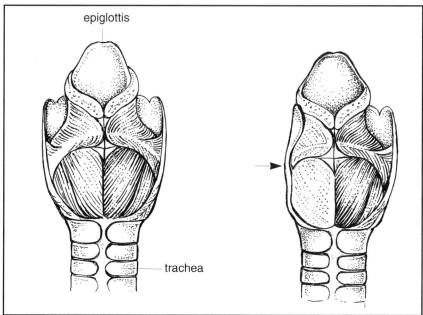

never been established. (Many horses make a noise after infection which passes off again.)

Right-sided paralysis is infrequent; up to 90 per cent of cases involve the left vocal cord.

As the paralysis develops, the cord loses its capacity to withdraw fully as air is inspired. This then forms a partial obstruction to the airflow and causes the abnormal sounds heard. To begin with, only a slight noise may be heard; this is described as a whistle, and is heard in a cantering horse when all four legs are off the ground, as it is filling its lungs with air. As the condition progresses, the noise becomes more pronounced in nature and deeper in volume and is then described as roaring. Along with this progression, the intimate condition of the larynx deteriorates with atrophy of muscles and distortion of the positioning of the arytenoid cartilage. A horse does not become a roarer first and a whistler later.

A slight whistle may not interfere significantly with performance, but the more advanced condition inhibits airflow to the lungs and prevents an animal from receiving adequate oxygen at faster paces.

Complicating Problems

When a horse is presented for examination, there may be a number of problems obscuring ILH. As any of these problems may lead to a false, or incorrect, diagnosis it is important to consider them here.

Any of the following may apply.

1)   Dorsal displacement of the soft palate. A horse suffering from DDSP will experience breathing problems which affect the intake of air.

The condition occurs when the soft palate is displaced upwards from its position under the epiglottis; in this position it creates turbulence in the path of incoming air, usually noted in the later stages of a race when air intake demands increase markedly. While the typical noise created by this is different from that in ILH, a rasping sound caused by the soft palate may confuse the picture and this may only be capable of being resolved through endoscopic examination.

2)   Bridle noises. When a horse is ridden or lunged with its head in a flexed position bridle noises may be heard.

The same may occur with dropped nosebands, which restrict airflow through the nostrils, or other faults - such as a fixed-head position - which are associated with bridle and bit.

It is vital to consider this when producing a horse for wind examination.

3)   Infections. Noises resulting from infections in the region of the pharynx, larynx, nasal passages and lungs often pass off again as the horse

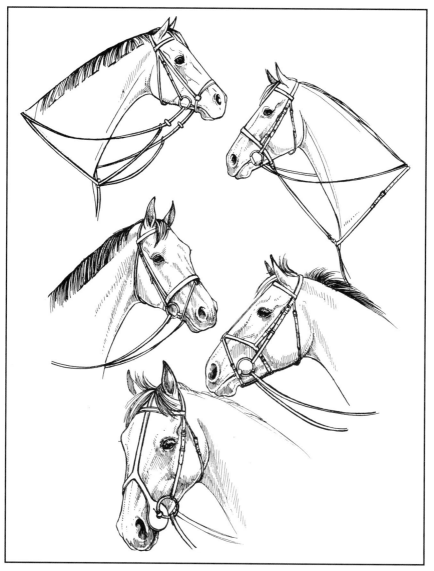

Different bridle restrictions. These may well have some effect on the horse's breathing: running and fixed martingales (top) *limit forward extension of the head; pressure of fitting over the nasal passages* (centre and bottom) *can create noises by restricting air intake*

recovers. The same applies to infection of the glands and related discharges. On endscopic examination the structures of the larynx may appear normal.

4)   Fat and unfit condition. Before any horse is subjected to a test for

Normal head position for a horse at exercise

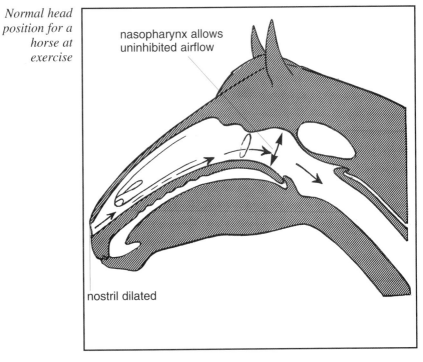

nasopharynx allows uninhibited airflow

nostril dilated

A fixed-head position may cause restriction of airflow in the pharangeal area; this may have an adverse influence on anatomical strutures as well as limiting air volume reaching the lungs

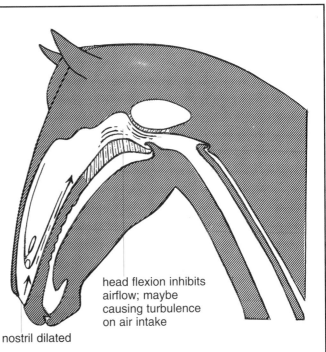

head flexion inhibits airflow; maybe causing turbulence on air intake

nostril dilated

its wind it is vital that it has been lunged or ridden for an adequate time in the days beforehand.

The horse should be capable of doing its exercise easily and without effort or resentment. Horses taken straight out of a field are placed under a strain and those which are fat and unfit may well fail to satisfy their examiner, only because it is not possible to subject them to an adequate exercise test.

Some such animals may make abnormal inspiratory noises which are not significant and which may never be heard again.

5)   High-blowers. Horses known as high-blowers make a characteristic noise when ridden. It is a noise produced by the horse on exhalation and is associated with the false nostril. It is in no way abnormal. Other noises which occur when an animal is exhaling are not usually significant.

Diagnosis

The diagnosis of ILH is achieved through physical examination at rest and during exercise, after which special tests may be undertaken. Examination of the wind is most frequently carried out by the vet as part of a general examination for soundness. However, in this situation, if an abnormal noise is heard, the animal would usually fail the test and no further examination would be undertaken.

The examination at rest will include evaluation of both the cardiac and respiratory systems, so that any abnormalities found here may be related to noises heard at exercise.

Where a noise is heard it is common to carry out an endoscopic examination of the larynx. This way the true condition of the vocal cords and related structures can be directly seen and assessed.

It needs to be appreciated that there are horses that make inspiratory noises in which performance is not affected; these noises often tend to become less marked as fitness increases. An objective assessment has to be made of ability to perform as well as consideration of any lesions found. It is equally true that some horses that appear abnormal under endoscopic examination are often able to perform unhindered.

Treatment

There is no non-surgical treatment for ILH. Various surgical operations are undertaken and have varying degrees of success. The older method involves stripping of the mucous membranes of the vocal cords - known as a Hobday operation, after the man who pioneered it. As the tissues heal

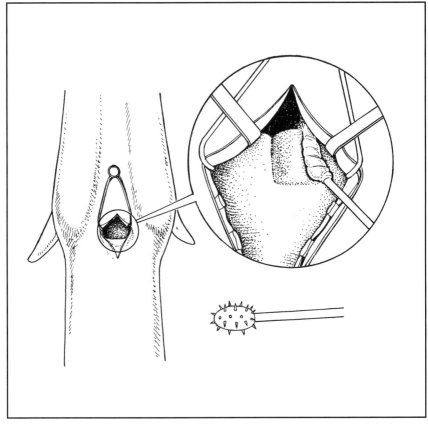

The Hobday operation. There is a mid-line incision (left)*; the lining of the horse's vocal cord is then stripped. In the latter part of the operation the veterinary surgeon employs a burr, a surgical instrument (*bottom, right)*, which is inserted into the incision and manipulated (*enlargement, right) *as part of the procedure*

the cord is drawn into close contact with the wall of the larynx. The Hobday operation, when performed before the condition has become too advanced, enjoys a fair measure of success.

Another surgical technique, the tie-back operation, involves restoring the shape of the larynx from outside its lumen. The mucous membrane of the vocal cord is normally stripped as well.

There is no way of preventing ILH although its incidence might be reduced if steps were taken to stop breeding from affected animals. In many countries stallions at stud are not licensed if they suffer from this condition. Unfortunately, however, this stipulation does not apply to

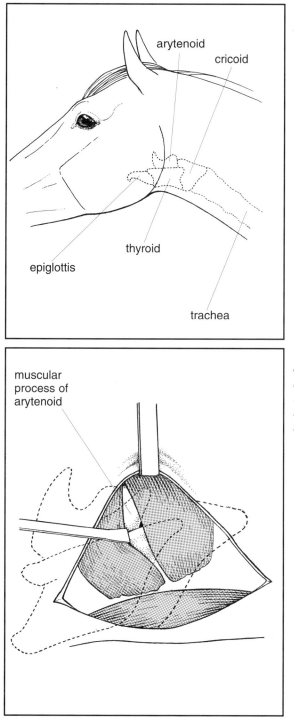

Tie-back operation: the position of the laryngeal cartilages relative to the surface

Tie-back operation: after the incision is made in the skin, muscle is retracted to expose the muscular process of the arytenoid

*Tie-back operation: the suture (stitch) attaches the muscular process of the arytenoid to the cricoid (*arrow*); the effect of this is to abduct the arytenoid and create a more natural anatomical shape to the larynx*

Tie-back operation: the skin wound has now been closed

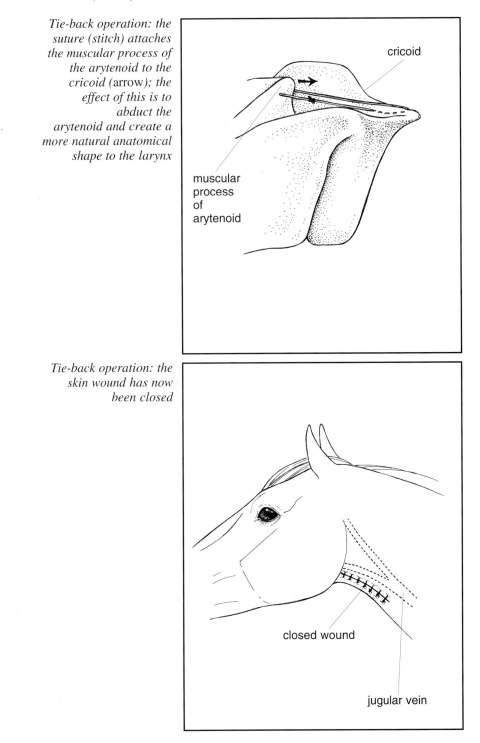

Thoroughbred breeding. The condition, it has to be said, is mainly one of larger horses and is uncommon in those animals under 16 hands high.

Palatopharyngeal Arch

Rostral displacement of the palatopharyngeal arch occurs when a fold of the mucous membrane at the back upper end of the pharynx overhangs the upper aspect of the larynx. This displacement may limit air intake.

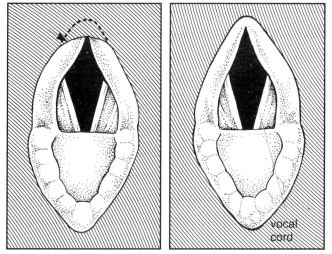

An endoscopic view of the normal larynx (near left); *and* (far left) *rostral displacement of the palatopharyngeal arch* (arrowed)

Epiglottic Entrapment

Epiglottic entrapment occurs when a fold of mucous membrane from beneath the epiglottis is sufficiently extensive to be able to rise over the front of the epiglottis and thus prevent its normal function of protecting the larynx.

In this condition, food material may enter the trachea, or, in extreme cases, the fold may be of sufficient length to inhibit air intake completely, especially towards the end of a gallop.

Soft Palate Displacement

Under normal conditions, the soft palate articulates (virtually) with the larynx and sits snugly around the epiglottis like a button-hole around a button.

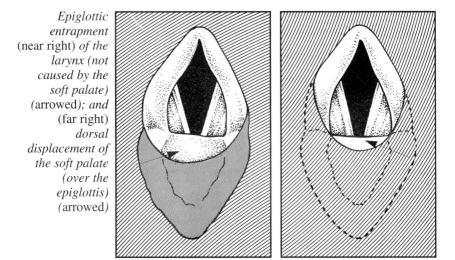

Epiglottic entrapment (near right) of the larynx (not caused by the soft palate) (arrowed); and (far right) dorsal displacement of the soft palate (over the epiglottis) (arrowed)

The design of this contact makes it exceptionally difficult for the horse to breathe through its mouth; this is the reason why vomited material is normally emitted through the nostrils. It is essential to normal breathing while racing (or competing) that the soft palate is unable to move above the epiglottis. Its displacement results in the condition known by the acronym, DDSP.

In DDSP there is an interference with airflow (usually at racing pace) and the animal may make a gurgling noise when it occurs. Such an occurrence will usually arise in the later part of a race, and diagnosis is confirmed by endoscopy. Some horses suffering from DDSP are said to 'swallow their tongue'; some will respond to having the tongue tied down, even with two separate ties. As this can prevent the tongue from pressing back against the epiglottis and displacing the soft palate upwards, the measure is met with a certain amount of success.

However, it must be appreciated that horses frequently make gurgling noises - especially in races when they are struggling for air. The reason for this may be the result of disease in the lungs as well as from anything that causes inadequate air intake. Many horses thus diagnosed as suffering from DDSP on the basis of this event alone will not benefit from having their tongue tied. The primary cause of the problem will need to be found and treated.

Severe Arytenoid Chondritis

The condition known as chondroma, or severe arytenoid chondritis is

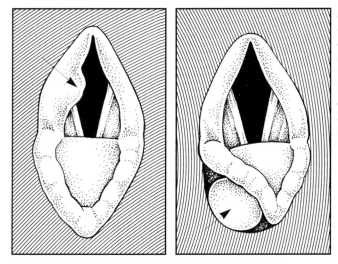

Endoscopic view of the larynx: arytenoid chondritis (far left) (arrowed); and (near left) subepiglottic cyst (arrowed)

caused by changes to the arytenoid cartilage itself. Such changes can be caused by tumour formation and narrowing of the laryngeal lumen.

Subepiglottic Cyst

Cyst formation underneath the epiglottis occurs on occasion and may cause upward displacement of the soft palate as well as moving the epiglottis itself upward into the laryngeal opening.

Diagnosis

All of these conditions are diagnosed by endoscope and are accepted as standard causes for rejection of horses at public sales in the United States.

In the United Kingdom and Ireland, ILH is usually the only condition for which sold horses can be returned as the situation stands at present.

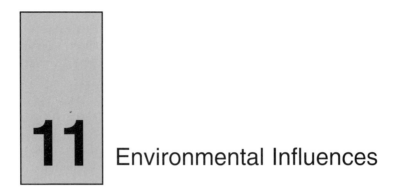

Environmental Influences

The horse's respiratory system is constantly influenced by environmental conditions whether it is kept outside at exercise, loose in a field, or indoors in its stable.

Outdoor Conditions

Keeping a horse outdoors subjects it not only to fluctuations of climate but also possible atmospheric pollution caused by chemicals or smoke from industrial and other sources. There is, too, the possibility of airborne infection or inhalation of organisms from the ground.

Breeds of horses vary in their ability to withstand these challenges: such variation will depend on thickness of skin, the protection of coats, and even the structure and strength of feet and so on. For example, the Thoroughbred and Arab horse are generally less robust animals than those native breeds of Scotland, Ireland, Wales and England and quite often have greater difficulty when out-wintered than do, say, moorland ponies.

The influences of snow and rain fall within the same parallels, being more testing for some than others; and it is normal to feed Thoroughbreds on concentrates when wintered outdoors, whereas native breeds are quite capable of sustaining themselves on lighter rations. Out-wintered Thoroughbreds are also often protected by New Zealand rugs, indicating appreciation of their need for warmth as well as their susceptibility to cold and disease.

Indoor Conditions

The competing animal is healthiest when kept indoors and in the correct environmental conditions. Infection is easier to control in such circumstances - though if the indoor environment is wrong the situation can be quite the reverse; returning infected horses to grass is sometimes the only path to take if good stabling conditions are not available, or if infection has built up to such a virulence that it cannot otherwise be controlled.

However, this does not always mean that horses are healthier outside, as horses at grass pick up just as many infections as those in stables. What is critical is the incidence and source of infection, the comings and goings that bring fresh organisms into a susceptible population.

Allergic conditions are caused by allergens, not stables; and infectious conditions are affected by poor stabling. Horses suffering from allergic respiratory conditions must therefore be kept away from the causative allergen as a first priority.

It is not the stable or the air-exchange that causes the condition to occur but an allergen; but stale, spore-laden atmospheres do exacerbate the symptoms and increase the demand for oxygen. If an animal has serious breathing problems, fresh air can be supplied without causing draughts. There is little logic in trying to create external conditions indoors which may only challenge the animal's resistance in another way and lead to infection on top of an allergy, further complicating the picture.

Horses are stabled for numerous management purposes, such as:

1)   Racing.
2)   Other competitive sports, such as showjumping, eventing, hunting, trotting.
3)   Stud purposes.
4)   Leisure riding.
5)   Working draft horses

Because the use of the animal is different in each case, individual requirements vary. The racehorse takes first place in this order because it demands higher standards of health care and disease prevention than any other horse. It has virtually no tolerance of respiratory disease while other breeds of horse can carry out their functions with at least a mild degree of impairment, because the workload allows it.

At stud, a different set of priorities exists because of the very nature of the business. The paralytic form of EHV-1 with abortion (and EVA now), is probably the most significant disease encountered in stud management, so much so that many modern building designs are intended to limit its virulence. As mares need to be housed for foaling, fertility inspection and protection from adverse weather conditions, the use of barns as an economic multi-purpose building has become almost standard.

However, the acknowledged risks of propagating infection has led to barns being excessively ventilated, which is sometimes a health risk in itself. The logic in this philosophy is the dilution of virus by increasing airflow, irrespective of whether or not this favours other infections.

In these circumstances, the opportunity arises for infective organisms to gain virulence and for mixed infections to occur because of multi-source congregation. While the inhibition of EHV-1 may appear, on the surface at least, beneficial, it cannot be denied that infection on large studfarms is a major problem that is nowhere close to control - low-grade infections are tolerated as long as they do not interfere with production and do not pose a threat to the life of mare or foal. That is, of course, with the solitary exception of EHV-1.

Stabling

The kind of information available on stabling today is, by and large, empirical. It is not information which is based on the solid foundation of scientific experiment but a collection of ideas which have over the years emanated largely from experience of disease. Often, such information is nothing more than opinion which might be less than objective; and quite frequently, it is patently wrong.

Trends have swayed in one direction or another, and few of these deserve to be treated as proven. Some ideas were derived from outbreaks of infection on studfarms; others are derived from experience in racing. However, in reaching conclusions, it appears to have been overlooked that requirements for, say, racehorses are essentially different from those for, say, broodmares.

For such opinions to be valuable they would have to be based on astute, objective observation, and a comprehensive understanding of disease. Sadly, this is not often the case and opinions are too often formed on error and misapprehension. Teaching, generally, has tended to follow fashion and, considering the importance of stabling in disease, this approach is no longer good enough.

The views expressed in this chapter are based on experience obtained within particular, significant disease outbreaks on studfarms and in racing. They are founded on trial and error and the pursuit of ideas influencing the spread of, and recovery from, disease which at first were nothing more than suspicions. However, they do provide a very strong basis for the treatment of sick horses, and offer a prospect of greater disease control if followed objectively. While these views are often at variance with modern convention, they do, by coincidence, agree with opinions expressed abundantly in earlier writing.

It has to be appreciated that every disease situation is different and also that the micro-climate of every building may vary; these realities have to be considered and any approach to disease control be conducted with objectivity.

Still, the expression of opinion does no more than contribute to the ongoing argument. Proof, on the other hand, is established by scientific trial carried out in a variety of situations. Considering the importance of the subject, it might be timely that some attention be given to it now, though there is little or no research being conducted presently.

A major aspect of indoor horse management is the relationship that exists between animal numbers and disease opportunity. In large yards, therefore, the essential elements that exist for creation of disease are:

1)   A susceptible population.
2)   Access to outside infection
3)   A confined area to allow build-up of organisms.

If there is considerable movement of animals in and out of a yard, then there is a possibility that infection may come from more than one source. And, if some buildings are so faulty in design that they are likely to precipitate disease, then the formula for trouble is completed.

Stable Environment

While the achievement of these ideals will depend on stable design and construction, it is the end product that is important to the health of the horse. Problems such as humidity, dampness, stale-smelling atmosphere, dust pollution, and so on, all need to be assessed as to cause and effect and then dealt with individually. Faults can often be corrected, although some stable designs are so badly flawed that they remain potential health risks by their very nature.

We look at some ideal requirements below.

Temperature Stability

Temperature stability, as an indoor environmental requirement, has been largely abandoned by modern equine management. Such an attitude is predominant in the stud scene and, when applied to horses in training, it considerably increases disease incidence. It also contributes to foal mortality in acute infectious outbreaks of disease.

As mentioned earlier in this book, the Victorian veterinarian W. J Miles was specific on temperatures (measured in degrees Fahrenheit):

'In summer 65 to 68 as a maximum, if possible, and in winter never below 50.' Also: 'It is desirable to have the stables sufficiently airy without cold or draught. It is taught in the old books that the horse, and the blood-horse especially, being originally denizens of a torrid country, require not only warmth but heat in this northern latitude.'

And, to conclude: 'The importance, then, of avoiding sudden and extreme alternations of heat and cold must be one of the points studied in the construction of a healthy stable.'

Fitzwygram, whom we also met earlier, advised that it was mistaken to use thermometers to gauge ideal indoor temperature requirements. This is, presumably, because excessively rigid adherence to thermometer readings might encourage ventilation errors.

Modern teaching is mistaken in tolerating far wider temperature ranges than those advised by Miles and Fitzwygram. While wider ranges are compatible with life, they encourage disease, especially in Thoroughbreds and can have a marked influence on the effectiveness of treatment in other breeds.

A Clean and Unpolluted Atmosphere

Both environmental purity and adequate air-exchange are inextricably tied together. They are, too, influenced not only by building design but also by management and hygiene as well as the type and quality of bedding used and the quality and cleanliness of feed - especially herbage. Avoiding air pollution is an essential aspect of management and depends as much on the selection of materials as exercising proper hygiene in their use.

Where inadequate air-exchange is a problem, this can usually be resolved by the adjustment of top-doors, vents and windows. There can also be positive air-extraction by means of mechanical fans. However, if the underlying cause of stale air is soiled bedding, the answer is to remove it and, where necessary, improve drainage.

Windows and vents when opened may need to be readjusted regularly to maintain temperature stability, depending on the prevailing external weather conditions. This requires application, observation and patience.

As we have already seen, the incidence of virus disease is higher than that of allergies or COPD, even though these latter conditions increase proportionally as animals grow older. As infectious diseases thrive on temperature instability it is not sensible to allow this for, say, the sake of reducing dust pollution. The answer to dust and allergens is equally important but separate, and should be treated as such, independently. It is not sensible to open all vents in order to live with sub-standard materials.

The persistence of atmospheric contamination after use of mouldy hay or straw is due to the spread of spores and other allergens onto mangers, walls, ceilings and even cobwebs. The natural answer to this is cleanliness and hygiene.

Condensation

Adequate air-exchange is dependent on the size of a building and the number of horses kept in it. If ventilation is inadequate there will often be condensation (from excessive humidity) as well as a rank humid smell.

Humidity is usually the result of air exhalation and the evaporation of excreta, but it may also reflect dampness in walls or inadequate insulation inside, say, tin roofs. The answer to condensation, smells and dampness is to remove the underlying cause, not simply to increase ventilation in a manner that will banish it but subject the animal to possible infection in the process. This means elimination of dampness in walls and floors by provision of a damp proof course. The elimination, too, of smells is achieved by greater attention to hygiene and by the provision of effective drainage.

The current cure for condensation is the installation of fixed open vents, often crudely broken through walls, thus solving one problem by creating another. Many modern stable units were originally built using breeze-blocks, and corrugated iron, or asbestos, roofing, without any insulation. In these units, condensation often became a major problem, causing cold water to drip onto horses. The easiest cure, instead of insulating the roof, was the introduction of fixed open ventilation at ridges, eaves and on gables. The condensation disappeared, but horses continued to suffer from respiratory disease.

Ventilation

Ventilation should always be discrete, and under control. The use of the word 'discrete' in this context means that any ventilation point should be of a size and design to suit a specific stable or stables. It should never amount to a hole knocked in a wall that cannot be blocked. Nor should it

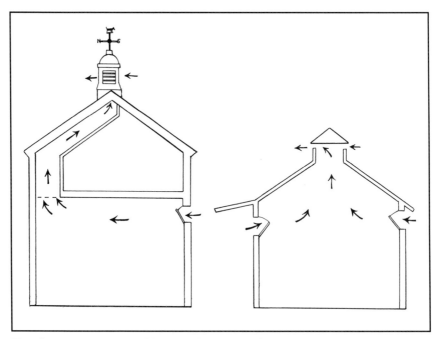

Ventilation systems: an older-style building (left) *with a discrete airflow system minimising draughts; a more modern-type building* (right) *with inlets on opposing walls, creating airflows which can cause disease in horses*

consist of a louvred vent which cannot be adjusted - or, indeed, will still let in air when it is supposedly shut. Control is all important.

It may be of interest here to point out that modern racing stables at Chantilly, and elsewhere in France, have ventilation only from the front door and overlying window - all adjustable. A small vent in the back of the ceiling allows the escape of foul air into the roof area.

Similarly, in multi-horse barns in Alpine areas on the Continent, insulation is total. Windows are double-glazed in most cases and the internal environment is warm but with clean air.

Design of stabling should therefore allow for no permanent open vents and any vents present should be fully adjustable and used to maintain temperatures even when conditions outside are fluctuating widely. It should be appreciated that temperatures can drop considerably during the night and supervising ventilation is a duty that requires constant care. When the horse is last attended to in the evening, therefore, it is critical to anticipate external changes; reducing ventilation may be necessary if the night is likely to become cold, and perhaps increasing it if a very warm night is expected. More thoughtfully-designed buildings have ventilation systems that operate effectively without constant supervision.

Inevitably, ventilation requirements vary between single stables and large buildings in which numbers of horses are kept. These requirements depend on the individual building, number of animals and the external conditions. Gauging these needs is often best done as a subjective exercise. If a groom feels cold in a stable, it is almost certain a horse will feel cold in it too. If it is too warm or humid, too stale or damp, these problems need to be corrected wisely.

Outlets and inlets need to be designed in such a way that they do not encourage draughts. Many older stable blocks provide evidence of the very different thinking of our ancestors on this subject. Some had simple extraction systems, based on a chimney principle, which allowed foul air to escape without exposing animals to excessive air-flows (i.e. warmth as well as air purity). Many of these systems are still to be seen today. Modern thinking, however, has very often left such systems closed and defunct, supplanted by permanent openings driven through external walls to relieve the condensation caused by this very change of thought.

In well-built single stables most air can be obtained from the front of the building (as in France), through the door or window. Foul air can escape at roof height, without any need for back wall vents or cross-flow between stables. While there may be an increased demand for airflow in warm weather, a well-insulated building will be cool in summer and warm in winter with no need for excessive supervision. A groom simply needs to appreciate the changes that occur in a twenty-four hour period and make allowance for them.

Airflows within a building for racehorses should be almost negligible, so as to be imperceptible. This does not mean, however, that if the atmosphere becomes rank the problem does not need to be resolved. But it should be done without creating draughts which would increase the risk of infection.

Insulation

Insulation is a first priority for controlling internal temperatures. This not only applies to walls and ceilings, but also to floors. In many cases, where floors are not insulated, the result is cold, humid air, damp, smelling beds, and the consequence is quite commonly intractable infection.

To achieve insulation of a stable, or a building used for stabling, it is essential, first, to use fully-insulated materials. Walls must be completely impermeable to rain, cold and damp. This will necessarily require the inclusion of a damp proof course (which is also vital in the construction of floors). Roofs and ceilings must also be fully insulated. Doors, vents and windows must be made of impervious material and properly sealed when closed. There should be no fixed open vents to the exterior of the building.

The influence dampness has on stable environment cannot be over-stressed. Uninsulated windows can contribute to damp by providing a cold surface against which condensation can form.

Drainage

The inevitable consequence of poor drainage in stables is wet and rank bedding. The influence of this on the stable environment is to increase humidity and pollute the atmosphere with ammonia. Both factors can and will contribute to disease.

Lying in wet surroundings is very unhealthy for horses and steps to improve drainage should be undertaken to avoid this situation.

Proper drainage is achieved by providing channels and by sloping floors in such a way that urine (and any other wet) is carried away from the horse to the exterior of the building in which it is housed. Underfloor drainage channels are useful, but can create smells and openings must be protected from blockage caused by loose bedding and litter and so on.

Stable Design

As this is not a book on stabling, this section will be confined to those aspects of stable design that influence disease. (Field shelters are not included.) More detailed advice on construction, materials and fittings can be obtained from other sources.

From a practical viewpoint, a horse owner must appreciate that the environment is an essential aspect of respiratory disease. However, this information is of more critical importance to the racehorse trainer than to the leisure rider, although all horses suffering respiratory disease will benefit from their owners' full appreciation of the environmental factors affecting their condition.

What this means in doing something to improve a poor building is that the basic needs for clean air and adequate warmth must be adhered to as far as is practical. Beds must be clean and any draughts eliminated if at all possible; adequate clean air must at all times be available especially for the acutely oxygen embarrassed horse.

High standards should be aimed at in constructing new stables; many of the prefabricated designs presently being marketed do not favour disease control.

Design requirements for construction of stabling are as follows.

1)   Single stable units (usually built in rows or back-to-back with others, or alternatively in squares or other designs). They should be built using materials that insulate them fully, with discrete ventilation control and no cross-flows of air.

Such units may be completely separate from each other, or linked over incomplete partitions. It is preferable that they be fully separated, as this has a critical influence on temperature control. Vents or peep-holes between boxes are a mistake; such arrangements are commonly found to be an influencing factor in disease. Uninsulated wooden stables are unsuitable housing for racehorses in training.

2)   Barns (available in a number of designs). The most common is a brick-built building with uninsulated roof and open ventilation at the eaves, ridge and on each gable. Some of the more modern buildings are

The inside of a modern barn. Many such buildings are inadequately insulated and excessively ventilated, thus aiding the communal development of disease. However, inadequate ventilation can be equally unhealthy especially if there is poor drainage and inadequate hygiene

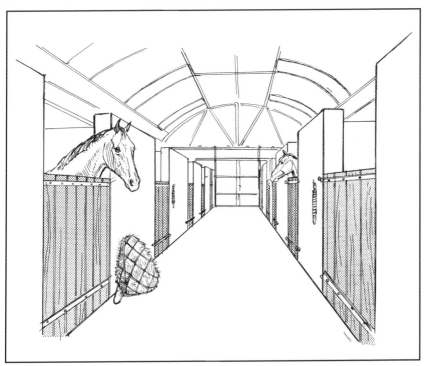

insulated, although there is a common mistaken tendency for fixed open vents on the walls.

Air extraction should be controlled and discrete. All inlets and outlets should be designed in a manner that limits excessive airflows. Open barns are a common influencing factor in infection.

3)   Separate loose-boxes in a common unit - the sort of accommodation in which the animal is not tied up. It needs to be big enough for the horse to be able to turn and lie down. The loose-boxes may be in sections, partitioned by walls often with bars at the front and on doors.

Many old yards were designed in this way and the style of ventilation system contained in most is a reflection of the current thinking at the time of their construction. While some of these buildings are ideal, others, for different reasons, are not. However, the basic concept was good, and many of these buildings can be a basis for incorporation into the better designs of the future.

A different style of loose-box within a modern barn. Railings between horses can influence airflow patterns, creating draughts and the risk of infection

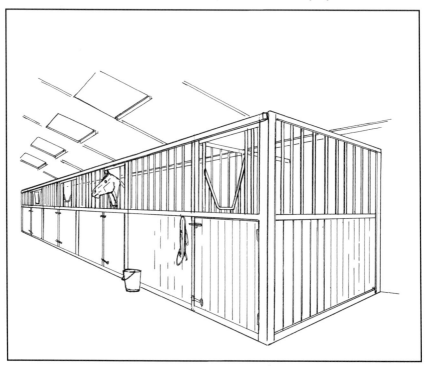

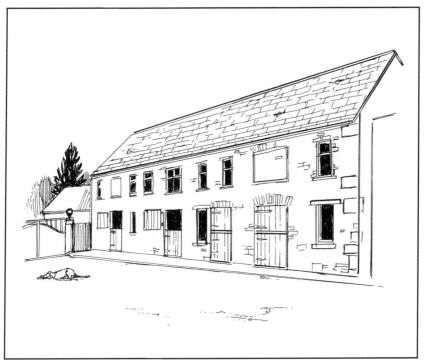

An old, lofted yard of individual stables. Damp walls and poorly-drained floors may be a feature of such buildings

Reasons for Stabling

The reasons for stabling horses are, of course, numerous. However, any design for stables will ensure the following:

1)   Control exercise fully.
2)   Control diet.
3)   Prevent injury.
4)   Simplify grooming.
5)   Limit disease.

To achieve these objectives, in addition to the disease control measures mentioned already in this, and earlier, chapters, the following will apply:

1)   The provision of a warm, dry bed in a clean atmosphere. While this topic has received considerable attention already, it does no harm to stress its importance as a first priority for the stabled horse.

2)   Good wholesome feeding provided through a system that will

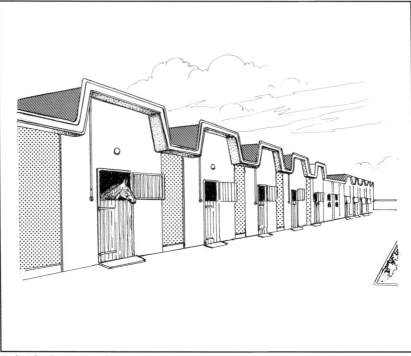

Individual, purpose-built boxes in a stallion yard. This type of design provides an individual environment for each animal and favours disease control

balance physical condition with exercise demand. Such a system of feeding will not allow for excess or deficiency.

3)   Under-floor insulation and correct drainage should ensure a dry place to lie.

4)   Bedding type should allow for minimal dust and dampness while providing adequate ground cover. The belief among many horse owners and grooms is that there is no substitute for clean, dust-free straw. However, good straw can be scarce in wet years and substitutes such as wood shavings, sawdust, peat and paper act as suitable alternatives. Wood shavings and sawdust are often naturally dusty when dry but settle down under proper management and are good forms of bedding when kept dry and clean. This, naturally, involves regular detailed attention. Peat provides bedding of a similar quality, but is often criticised for the dirty appearance it creates.

The main criticism of paper is the poor ground cover it provides when fresh and the problems of providing a clean, dry bed with it when deep-littered. Paper is, however, often the bedding of choice where horses suffer from COPD.

5)   Hay quality should be high in nutrient value and free of dust; an alternative should be used if these requirements cannot be met. Haylage is a grass product that often acts as a suitable alternative for horses on a dust-free diet. It is cut when green, chopped, wilted and stored in an air-tight manner, either in bags or, possibly, in special tower silos. Good quality silage, stored in air-tight bags, is also increasingly used today. While care needs to be taken of quality and conditions under which it is fed, it can prove a suitable feed, especially for hunters. It is especially important to avoid samples that have been exposed to air and on which moulds have formed. It is also critical to introduce horses to this type of feeding on a gradual basis.

6)   Where possible, dust should only be created when the horse is out of its stable. This applies to shaking out beds and also to dusting down walls, ceilings and partitions.

7)   Gauge the ventilation requirements of the horse in an objective manner, taking into consideration the comments expressed earlier in this chapter. In buildings which tend to be hot and humid at evening stables, remember to allow for night-time temperature fluctuations; thus vents and windows may need to be adjusted regularly as your horse cannot escape from the environment within the stable, even when this changes radically during the night. The answer is not to get out of bed, but to use discretion when last seeing the horse in the evening.

8)   The cure for dampness is insulation. Very often, this can be done economically, using plastic or foam materials. There are many materials available for damp-proofing walls, but do not forget floors, as these may be the cause of dampness and may contribute to disease.

9)   The answer to humidity is correct extraction. Many different types of extractor are available today, some solar operated and functionally effective in large buildings. Needless to say, they should not act as air inlets when not working. Electrical extractors placed in the roof of a large building will extract foul air and can be set to work on a timed basis. It must be remembered, however, that extraction of air from a stable does not have to be done by mechanical extractors. Warm air rises and can escape through ceiling or roof outlets, but it is important that these outlets do not act as entry points for cold air. It is also vital to humidity control in stables that beds are clean and dry and that their condition is not allowed to unduly influence air pollution.

10)   Never subject horses to draughts. For the ordinary horse owner, the control of draughts may be less critical than for a racehorse trainer, but

the principles are the same. If there is no outlet for air on the back wall of the stable, so much the better.

Incomplete partitions between stables can be easily closed with wood or plastic but must be sealed at the edges (inevitably, neither material is suitable if capable of being eaten by horses, but can be effective when out of reach).

Improperly fitting doors and windows are another obvious source that may have an undesirable effect on horses' health, especially during the colder months of the year. Never have open ridges or eaves in stables for competing horses.

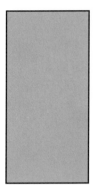

Index